T0233434

A clinico-genetic study of psychiatric disorder in Huntington's chorea

Huntington's chorea (HC) is a dominantly inherited neurological disorder of movement accompanied by dementia. It is progressive, leading to severe disability in five to ten years and death within a further ten. In the course of the illness, and sometimes before the onset of organic symptoms, periods of functional psychiatric disorder (fpd) of varying types occur; these add to the burden of the illness and of caring for affected subjects. An opportunity of examining these conditions was provided in 1983 by a discovery that enabled a genetic test to be developed. This test brought to genetic departments young adult couples who were contemplating marriage or procreation, where one adult from each couple was from an HC family, seeking information about the test. These young adults were more numerous and provided a more open and informative attitude about their family than had formerly been the case. This gave an enhanced opportunity, facilitating the examination of a larger number of affected subjects and their unaffected relatives.

A detailed description of the genetic basis of HC and of the test is given here. The incidence of diagnostic categories of fpd is compared for affected HC subjects with subjects of 50% initial risk of HC, with subjects of zero risk in a similar environment, with subjects affected with long-standing, disabling, incurable disease and, for those who by pre-symptomatic genetic testing are shown to be carrying the HC gene, with those in whom it is shown to be absent. The interval between the onset of organic symptoms of HC and the onset of fpd was measured and the bearing of all these results on the relation of HC to fpd is discussed, together with the future prospects of the genetics of HC.

Psychological Medicine

David C. Watt and Anneke Seller

A clinico-genetic study of psychiatric disorder in Huntington's chorea

MONOGRAPH SUPPLEMENT 23

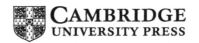
CAMBRIDGE
UNIVERSITY PRESS

CAMBRIDGE UNIVERSITY PRESS
Cambridge, New York, Melbourne, Madrid, Cape Town, Singapore,
São Paulo, Delhi, Dubai, Tokyo, Mexico City

Cambridge University Press
The Edinburgh Building, Cambridge CB2 8RU, UK

Published in the United States of America by Cambridge University Press, New York

www.cambridge.org
Information on this title: www.cambridge.org/9780521459839

© Cambridge University Press 1993

First published 1993

A catalogue record for this publication is available from the British Library

ISBN 978-0-521-45983-9 Paperback

CONTENTS

List of Tables

List of Figures

This study was supported by grants from the Wellcome Trust and the Huntington Disease Association and carried out in collaboration with Professor J. E. Edwards, with the cooperation of Dr R. Lindenbaum and Dr S. Huson. Clinical data were collected by Dr R. Shiwach with assistance from Mrs Annona Galliard. Data from the case register were retrieved with the help of Dr E. Rosser. Mrs Gail Norbury assisted with the genetic linkage analysis. Miss W. Ashman and Mrs Peggy Ducker typed and word-processed drafts of the manuscript.

LIST OF TABLES

LIST OF FIGURES

SYNOPSIS   The introduction in 1985 of a genetic linkage test programme to identify asymptomatic heterozygotes among subjects at 50% initial risk for Huntington's chorea[1] required a review of all cases of Huntington's chorea and their families referred to the Department of Medical Genetics of the Oxford Regional Health Area (population 2·5 million). From a representative sample of these subjects, psychiatric data were collected to estimate the frequency and time of onset of functional psychiatric illness and behaviour disorder. The rationale and method of the linkage test is described. The frequency of functional psychiatric disorder found was compared with that reported for the general population and for Alzheimer's disease. The role in relation to the aetiology of functional psychiatric disorder (1) of the Huntington's chorea gene and (2) of the family disturbance produced, was investigated by comparison between the frequency of functional psychiatric disorder in populations containing different proportions of heterozygotes as shown by (a) the manifestation of Huntington's chorea, and (b) the result of the genetic linkage analysis. In order to investigate the influence of the onset of Huntington's chorea on the production of functional psychiatric disorder the time of onset of the various functional psychiatric disorders was compared between asymptomatic subjects at 50% risk for Huntington's chorea and their cohabiting spouses who were assumed to be at at zero risk and who shared their environment. It is concluded that possessing the Huntington's chorea gene: (1) has no influence on the production of functional psychiatric disorder in asymptomatic subjects at risk for Huntington's chorea; and (2) increases the tendency to major depressive disorder in subjects already affected with physical signs of Huntington's chorea.

---

[1] Usually referred to as Huntington's Disease in the USA since 1975.
Address for correspondence: Dr David C. Watt, 7 Churchway, Stone, Aylesbury, Bucks. HP17 8RG.

Chapter 1

Introduction

The opening paragraph of Caine & Shoulson's (1983) study of psychiatric syndromes in Huntington's chorea states that 'Huntington's disease presents a unique opportunity to investigate the development and evolution of psychopathological disorders. As a fully penetrant genetic disorder that can be diagnosed with great certainty, it provides an investigative setting seldom available to researchers studying "functional" psychiatric syndromes. The presence of an abnormal movement disorder and a positive family history provide "external" validating factors. Certain diagnosis is not in question.' The cogency and relevance of this statement has been reinforced by the advent of a test for distinguishing the presence of the gene for Huntington's chorea in asymptomatic carriers (Gusella *et al.* 1983). The present study is an attempt to take this opportunity.

1.1 HUNTINGTON'S CHOREA

Sydenham in 1686 distinguished chorea from other movement disorders (Sydenham 1848–1850) and about two hundred years later, in 1872, Huntington separated a sub-group of chorea, now named after him, by distinguishing four definitive features. It is hereditary, progressive, has an onset in adult life and 'shows a tendency to insanity'. Cerebral pathology, subsequently added to these features, was slowly delineated but not established as a diagnostic factor, by Dunlap, until 1927. It has the advantage of being diagnostically unequivocal, but was accessible only by post mortem examination until recent methods of imaging were introduced. As with most genetic diseases during this period there was little opportunity for therapeutic intervention and effort was directed towards assessing the scope of the problem and its public health implications, as indicated by the considerable number of epidemiological studies of Huntington's chorea in which a population exceeding 1 million was surveyed (Panse, 1942; Bell, 1948; Pearson *et al.* 1955; Kishimoto, 1957; Parker, 1958; Read & Chandler, 1958;

Wendt *et al.* 1959; Heathfield, 1968; Bolt, 1970; Wallace, 1972; Wallace & Parker, 1973; Myrianthopoulos, 1973; Mattsson, 1974*a*; Stevens, 1976; Harper, 1979; Hayden *et al.* 1980; Walker *et al.* 1981). These constantly give evidence of the 'tendency to insanity' which made such a strong impression on the young George Huntington whose father and grandfather had studied the same families.

1.2 PATHOLOGY

Huntington's chorea is a dominant hereditary degeneration of the brain, prominently of the basal ganglia but also affecting the cortex and other parts. It manifests usually in middle-age with chorea, progressive cognitive impairment and emotional and behaviour disorder. There is no effective treatment and death occurs in about 15 years. Macroscopic examination of the brain shows marked atrophy of the caudate nucleus with dilatation of the lateral ventricles, particularly of their frontal horns. This appearance is characteristic and its presence provides the most reliable confirmation of the diagnosis of Huntington's chorea in a family. It is reflected in the CAT and PET scans which, however, are not sufficiently specific for diagnosis (Neophytides *et al.* 1979; Hayden *et al.* 1987*a*) and cannot replace post mortem examination. Histology shows extensive loss of neurons in the striatum and in the cortex of the frontal and parietal lobes which results in massive abnormalities of brain and the neurotransmitter concentrations of receptors (Marsden, 1982).

The onset of Huntington's chorea is insidious and although suspected at an early stage may be too uncertain to allow diagnosis (Myers *et al.* 1984).

1.3 PSYCHIATRIC DISORDER IN HUNTINGTON'S CHOREA

An important constituent of psychiatric disorder in Huntington's chorea is cognitive impairment, a component of the organic syndrome directly attributable to cerebral pathology. The most striking psychiatric features, however, show characteristics indistinguishable from those of functional psychiatric disorders, the major psychoses, neuroses, personality and behaviour disorders. These contribute to the frequent picture of social catastrophe so striking to observers having direct contact with affected families. Thus, Oliver & Dewhurst (1969) illustrating from a pedigree of six generations 'representative of many others studied in depth involving at least 425 families', in which 'children from at least four generations were subjected to both active cruelty and passive neglect', cite an affected individual '...always in rages and tempers...vicious and cruel to all her children'; a man in his 40s who, before the clear onset of Huntington's chorea, was 'out of work, depressed, and under the impression that his wife was being persistently unfaithful to him... and had irrational aggressive outbursts against his wife and children, but otherwise showed little interest in his children, who were frequently farmed out to mentally-sick relatives'; a woman who followed 'a feckless existence of casual prostitution starting a line of problem families, delinquents and jailbirds'; 'a man whose worklessness, physical violence, headaches and insomnia...drove his wife to leave him, abandoning their child to the care of unwilling grandparents who in turn farmed him out to a psychotic aunt'. Although the emphasis in this paper is on physical abuse of children, it also gives instances of children's abuse of parents and aggression, suspicion and indifference towards spouses. The authors point out that mental instability also appears in spouses not at risk for Huntington's chorea and in blood relatives showing no physical signs of Huntington's chorea. For instance, in one generation of 20 individuals (all offspring of affected parents), in which three are affected with Huntington's chorea, four of the unaffected showed mental illness and the wife of an affected man 'had a bitter and sadistic temperament' exemplified during visits to her son in gaol or in a special hospital, when 'she discussed either his wife's infidelities or details of his father's perversions'.

1.4 SURVEYS OF FUNCTIONAL PSYCHIATRIC DISORDER IN HUNTINGTON'S CHOREA

Seven surveys of functional psychiatric disorder in Huntington's chorea are summarized in Table 1. The figures shown have been derived from those supplied in the studies and where necessary converted to percentage frequencies to facilitate comparisons. Functional illness is shown separately from personality and behaviour disorder. The frequencies range from 21 to 56% for functional illness and from 24 to 70% for personality and behaviour disorder. This variation must be partly a product of the different diagnostic criteria employed and of the different arrangements and circumstances of the surveys. The authors obtaining low figures for illness (Hughes, Bolt, Mattson, Saugstad) deal only with psychosis while the remainder include neuroses and personality disorder (Dewhurst) or 'psychiatric disturbance' (Wallace). The explanation of the low figure of Saugstad & Ødegård (1986) for psychiatric illness is that it includes only the single diagnosis made during first psychiatric admission, before Huntington's chorea was diagnosed.

Mattsson employs three diagnoses only: (1) depressive-anxious state; (2) schizophrenic-paranoic state; and (3) personality disorders. Personality changes and behaviour disorders are described in a comprehensive list of 23 morbid behaviours, offences and attitudes by Hughes (1925), but Wallace (1972) limits himself to two: 'anger outbursts'; and 'sexual aberration'. The only survey using standardized diagnosis is Folstein *et al.* (1983*a*) who employ DSM-III, with the added condition that major depression must have lasted at least a month to be diagnosed.

We must question whether estimates of prevalence have been taken from epidemiological samples, i.e. samples which include all subjects showing the disease within a specified area at a specified time. Samples including only hospital admissions leave out patients who have not been admitted. For those that include deceased subjects it must be decided whether these subjects were living and affected in the specified area at the specified time. To allow generalization, the diagnosis must arise from agreed descriptions, preferably using standardized diagnostic pro-

Table 1. *Proportion of functional psychiatric disorder found in 7 surveys of Huntington's chorea*

Author	Location	Population surveyed	Number of affected HC subjects (N)	Criteria for specifying functional psychiatric disorder	Circumstances of making diagnosis of functional psychiatric disorder	Stages of Huntington's chorea included in N	Functional psychiatric illness (%)	Personality and behaviour disorder (%)
Hughes (1925)	Michigan, USA	Institutionalized cases and their affected kin	218	Clinical diagnosis from hospital records and personal interview	Cases presenting behaviour problems after development of Huntington's chorea	All stages; dead included	27 (of 175 cases with data available)[1]	70 (after chorea)[2]
Dewhurst *et al.* (1969)	Great Britain	Cases in 5 neighbouring counties	92	Author's retrospective clinical diagnosis from records and survey history	Diagnosis during first admission to a psychiatric hospital	All stages	40[3]	Not ascertained
Bolt (1970)	W. Scotland	11 western counties Pop. 2·96 m	334	Summary of clinical features from hospital records. Clinical diagnosis	Functional psychosis noted as on admission	All stages; dead included	26[4]	59 (clinical features)
Wallace (1972)	Queensland, Australia	Survey of Queensland Pop. 1·75 m	182	Clinical diagnosis from author's examination	Survey discovered history or presence of psychiatric disorder	All stages; all living	56[5]	47 (anger and sexual aberration)
Mattsson (1974*b*)	Sweden	Survey of Swedish institutions admitting Huntington's chorea	162	Choice of 3 diagnoses made from clinical records	Diagnosis on first admission to a psychiatric hospital	All stages from admission to psychiatric hospital; dead included	32[6]	24 (initial diagnosis)
Saugstad & Ødegård (1986)	Norway	National psychiatric register, 1st admissions for 60 years. Pop. 3·28 m	229	Clinical diagnosis recorded in national psychiatric register	Diagnosis during first admission to a psychiatric hospital	All stages from admission to psychiatric or neurological unit; dead included	21[7]	56 (personality disorder prior to admission)
Folstein *et al.* (1986)	Maryland, USA	Population survey. Pop. 4·2 m	186	DSM-III (1980) from interview and records (modified for major depression)	All living affected Maryland subjects examined by authors up to the date of survey	All stages; all living	47[8]	37 (explosive and personality disorder)

Alcoholism has not been included. This material is derived from the following in the publications: [1] Table 7; [2] p. 550; [3] p. 256(*e*); [4] p. 256(*e*); [5] Appendix; [6] Table 10; [7] Table 3; [8] Table 6.

cedures. Bolt (1970) makes an estimate of prevalence from a representative sample which is not, however, the sample on which her observations on functional psychiatric disorder are based. Of those appearing in Table 1, only the study of Wallace can be considered to have based the estimate of the prevalence of Huntington's chorea on an epidemiological sample. The excellent study of Folstein is unfortunately marred by a curious error of ascertainment. Subjects ascertained after the day on which prevalence was estimated, but who were living in the specified area and affected on that day, were not included in the prevalence estimates (Folstein, 1989, p. 90). Overall, it is estimated that functional illness results in $\frac{1}{3}$ to $\frac{1}{2}$, and personality and behaviour disorder in $\frac{1}{4}$ to $\frac{2}{3}$, of affected subjects.

Despite the variation in amount, all these surveys show a substantial frequency of psychiatric illness identified as such by psychiatrists, and a larger amount of seriously disordered behaviour which is often disruptive of family life and at times results in legal process and imprisonment. The study of Saugstad & Ødegård (1986) indicates the large number of affected persons admitted to a psychiatric hospital with psychosis before Huntington's chorea manifested itself. (Table 1) by physical signs.

In accounting for the variety of results obtained from these studies, three elements in the method have become apparent. The first is the period in the course of Huntington's chorea at which the subject is studied. The course can be divided into: (1) pre-choreic; (2) early; and (3) late stages, varying proportions of which may be represented in the populations studied. The second element arises from the frequent use of psychiatric hospital contact as a convenient method of collecting information about a population of Huntington's choreics. Here the events recorded at the out-patient attendance or at first admission are most frequently used, but stages in the course of the hospital stay may be defined, such as cause of admission, and information taken from these as in Dewhurst *et al.* (1969). Finally, the criteria used for identifying the functional disorder may be chosen by the investigator as most appropriate for the material found (e.g. Mattsson, 1974*a*) or the diagnosis recorded in the hospital records may be adopted (Dewhurst *et al.* 1969) or a standardized di-

agnostic system may be used, such as the DSM-III, as in Folstein (1989).

1.5 TYPES OF FUNCTIONAL PSYCHIATRIC DISORDER IN HUNTINGTON'S CHOREA

The types and proportions of functional psychiatric disorder found in Huntington's chorea are shown for two complete systematic studies in Table 2. Both studies are population surveys

Table 2. *The diagnoses of functional psychiatric disorder in two populations of subjects with Huntington's chorea*

Symptom or syndrome	Bolt* (%)	Folstein† (%)
Depression	32	33
Schizophrenia	—	6
Paranoid delusions	33	—
Irritability, rage	51	36
Personality change	8	6
N	334	186

* Bolt (1970) – Table 4.
† Folstein *et al.* (1987) – Table 6.

in which living persons affected with Huntington's chorea within a limited region were ascertained and examined by the authors. The majority of cases in both studies had previously been admitted to hospital or were resident. In Folstein's study the diagnoses conform to DSM-III criteria (APA, 1980), but in Bolt's study diagnoses are taken from hospital reports and the population is enlarged by the addition of the clinical records of deceased affected relatives of the index cases she contacted. In both studies, therefore, patients in all stages of the illness are included with, as Folstein (1989) points out, a possible under-representation of manifestations with onset in the course of late-onset Huntington's chorea. Differences of method between the two studies will account for some of the difference in results, but nevertheless the proportion of depression and of irritability and rage is high in both studies. The lower proportion of irritability and rage in Folstein *et al.* (1987) is probably attributable to the criterion for this feature being the DSM-III category 'Intermittent explosive disorder' which requires that the episode results in 'serious assault or destruction of property'. Bolt applies the diagnosis schizo-phrenia (and paranoid psychosis) only to mis-diagnoses attributed early in the course of Huntington's chorea. Categories of illness resembling schizophrenia occurring throughout the course of Huntington's chorea are contained within her category 'paranoid delusions', which shows a striking difference in frequency (33%) from Folstein *et al.*'s 'Schizophrenia' (6%), the low figure probably attributable to their adherence to DSM-III as criterion.

1.6 STAGES OF HUNTINGTON'S CHOREA AT WHICH FUNCTIONAL PSYCHIATRIC DISORDER OCCURS

The observation that functional psychiatric disorder is frequent in the early, even pre-choreic, period of Huntington's chorea (Matt-sson, 1974*b*: Folstein, 1989), often leading to misdiagnosis (Bolt, 1970; Mattsson, 1974*b*; Saugstad & Ødegård (1986) raises the question of the stages of the illness at which functional psychiatric disorder occurs. First admission to a psychiatric hospital is the most frequently quoted stage of illness for showing the extent and composition of functional psychiatric disorder. It is the most conspicuous event in professional recognition of the illness and is the first occasion on which the diagnosis is administratively recorded and dated. Mattsson (1974*b*) observes that initial symptoms are psychiatric in about half of the cases and that disorders of consciousness (confusional states) are never seen. Dewhurst *et al.* (1969) list 'prodromal symptoms', which they observe are non-specific and would not by themselves suggest Huntington's chorea. Presenting symptoms at the onset of the disease were psychiatric in well over half of their 102 cases. They stress that 'these syndromes are not separate entities; they merely reflect a preponderance of signs and symptoms rather than a distinct classification', thus emphasizing the difficulty of assigning a formal psychiatric diagnosis over the whole range of the functional psychiatric disorders seen in Huntington's chorea. Dewhurst *et al.* (1969) give the proportions of different types of functional disturbance that they found at four stages: in the prodromal period, among the earliest presenting symptoms, among the reasons for admission to a psychiatric hospital and among the diagnoses made at first admission. They draw attention to the many patients 'wrongly regarded as having a psychiatric illness *per se* owing to the fact that several signs and symptoms would equally well substantiate a psychiatric or neurological diagnosis'.

The retrospective observation from studies of affected subjects that functional psychiatric disorder sometimes has its onset before the onset of Huntington's chorea makes it mandatory that those at risk and still asymptomatic should be examined, as well as affected subjects, to make a complete assessment of the stage of Huntington's chorea at which functional psychiatric disorder occurs.

1.7 FUNCTIONAL PSYCHIATRIC DISORDER AS AN INDICATION OF LIABILITY TO HUNTINGTON'S CHOREA IN SUBJECTS AT AN INITIAL 50% RISK

In earlier studies of Huntington's chorea (Davenport & Muncey, 1916; Hughes, 1925) the occurrence of functional psychiatric disorder in the pre-morbid period attracted investigators' attention because it might indicate which relatives of an affected person at an initial 50% risk would themselves develop the disease. Hughes (1925) reports that during the pre-morbid period of 172 affected cases 'temperamental irregularities' stood out markedly in 42%. The author cites easily excited, shrewish, inconsistent, seclusive, stubborn, and uninhibited display of eroticism, as examples. Hughes found, however, that 32% of the known cases had not displayed any such disturbance and that 'all of the traits recorded in those who became choreic were found in their non-choreic relatives'. Her conclusion agrees with that of Davenport & Muncey (1916) that 'there is no universal symptom indicating which member of a fraternity will develop chorea'.

1.8 CATEGORIZATION OF FUNCTIONAL PSYCHIATRIC DISORDER IN HUNTINGTON'S CHOREA

Considerable differences between authors are shown in the criteria of diagnosis used in categorizing the functional psychiatric disorders found in Huntington's chorea. Many authors rely on the diagnosis found in medical records of hospital admission which follows customary psychiatric hospital nosology (Hughes, 1925; Bolt, 1970; Wallace, 1972; Mattsson, 1974 *b*). Dewhurst *et al.* (1969) searched records of 88 patients from a group of neighbouring mental hospitals for evidence of functional psychiatric disorder and differentiated their description according to stages of patients' stay in hospital, for instance, prodromally and on admission, in terms of current psychiatric hospital nosology; the 'reason for admission' in terms of prominent features which are socially disabling or disturbing; the course in hospital in terms of symptoms classified as affective or psychotic features. Folstein *et al.* (1979), noted that most previous reports of psychiatric symptomatology in Huntington's chorea were subjective and therefore used standardized and validated diagnostic methods to quantify more precise clinical categories in a group of 11 affected subjects. All 11 patients showed detectable functional psychiatric disorder, most of which was severe. Only five of the 11 subjects, however, were given formal diagnosis, while the remainder were categorized as hallucinatory state, anxious, demoralized, irritable or withdrawn. All 11 patients, only two of whom gave measurable evidence of dementia, therefore showed detectable functional psychiatric disorder, most of which was severe, but less than half could be categorized in a standardized diagnostic scheme. A considerable difference was shown from the same unit in the results of a survey of functional psychiatric disorder in Huntington's chorea in the general population of Maryland (Folstein *et al.* 1987). DSM-III was again used and 90% of functional psychiatric disorders were diagnosed without recourse to the symptomatic description employed by Folstein *et al.* (1979) described above.

1.9 TYPES OF FUNCTIONAL PSYCHIATRIC DISORDER

1.9.1. Depression

Depression is frequently noted in practically all surveys of psychiatric disturbance in Huntington's chorea (Davenport & Muncey, 1916; Dewhurst *et al.* 1969; McHugh & Folstein, 1975; Caine & Shoulson 1983; Folstein *et al.* 1983*c*, 1987). Folstein (1989) describes depressive illness as the most common psychiatric

syndrome seen early in Huntington's chorea. The features reported are those encountered in the general population as are the varied forms in which depression appears and its greater frequency among women (Tamir *et al.* 1969; Bolt, 1970).

In the Maryland survey encompassing 217 cases of Huntington's chorea, Folstein and colleagues (1983*c*) have given particular attention to affective disorder. From each of 186 persons with Huntington's chorea a medical history was compiled and examination, which included a DSM-III (APA, 1980) psychiatric examination and showed that 38% had a history of major affective disorder or dysphoria (painful emotion), a larger proportion than for any other psychiatric category. Reactive depression was sharply distinguished and separated from major affective disorder. Chronic depression (under 5%) and mania were infrequent.

1.9.2 Schizophrenia

In the period during which functional psychiatric disorder has been observed in Huntington's chorea, two important changes have occurred in making the diagnosis of schizophrenia. The first is that whereas paranoid disorders were formerly thought to be distinct from schizophrenia, with a small area of overlap, they are now combined under the term schizophrenia, with the exception of the rare condition true paranoia. The clear adoption of this view in the first edition of the textbook of Mayer-Gross *et al.* (1954) was an early indication of this change. Thus, Bickford (1953) gives 9/19 (47%) cases of Huntington's chorea with 'paranoid delusions' from a population of 341 000; Bolt (1970) gives the prevalence of 'schizophrenia' in 334 cases derived from hospital records as 2% and paranoid psychosis as 15% whereas Folstein *et al.* (1982) found a total of 5–9% schizophrenia (p. 174, Table 6). Dewhurst *et al.* (1969), reporting different stages of the course of Huntington's chorea, give 2% of all functional psychiatric disorders (68) as paranoidal delusional states in the prodromal stage and, as initial diagnosis, schizophrenia (18%). Interestingly, the estimates of Folstein and her colleagues vary from 1979, no schizophreniza and 18% 'hallucinatory states' who did not meet all research criteria for schizophrenia, to 1987, 5·9% schizophrenia which the authors point out may be an underestimate, and no other schizophrenia-like diagnosis.

The second change is the adoption of standardized criteria of diagnosis in psychiatric examination. The effect of this procedure on the diagnosis of schizophrenia has been to narrow the range of psychopathology included within the diagnosis of schizophrenia leaving an increased residue labelled as 'schizophrenia symptoms'. These difficulties with schizophrenia are again illustrated by the Baltimore Huntington Disease Project where, in the course of the following five reports, subjects are labelled as (1) 'delusional-hallucinatory', indistinguishable from schizophrenia, but not identical with it (McHugh & Folstein, 1975); (2) 'hallucinatory state', which many psychiatrists would call schizophrenia but which did not meet all research criteria and did not respond to phenothiazines (Folstein *et al.* 1979); (3) 'hallucinosis', sometimes called schizophrenia, noticeably in mental hospital case records in the absence of clear delusions, which may have been suppressed by halperidol prescribed for chorea (Folstein & Folstein, 1983); (4) 'delusionary and hallucinatory states', particularly in young women where schizophrenia may have appeared before dementia and then been obscured by it (Folstein & McHugh, 1983); and finally, (5) schizophrenia was diagnosed in 10 Huntington's disease patients in 8 years of observation (Folstein, 1989). The latter used standardized diagnosis (DSM-III-R, APA, 1987) of functional psychiatric disorder in Huntington's chorea, but it is evident from them that standardized diagnostic procedures exclude a considerable amount of clinical material which, if it cannot be subsumed under schizophrenia, cannot be included in any other diagnostic category.

1.9.3 Prechoreic cases

A number of patients are admitted to psychiatric facilities and diagnosed as schizophrenia who are later diagnosed as Huntington's chorea. Streletski (1961) reviewed 1200 adequately recorded cases of Huntington's chorea in a review of case records in Germany (quoted in Slater & Cowie, 1971). Among these were 32 (3%) cases of schizophrenia (including paranoid states) which occurred early in the illness. Markowe and colleagues (1967) reported a 10-year follow-up of 100 hospitalized schizophrenics. Nine

died, of whom one was found on autopsy to have Huntington's chorea. Two consultants had agreed the diagnosis of schizophrenia, on which they had no doubt. Saugstad & Ødegård (1986) had National Case Register information for Norway, from which they reported 199 psychiatric first admissions of subjects with Huntington's chorea. Of these 39 left hospital with a discharge diagnosis of schizophrenia or paranoid psychosis only. Huntington's chorea was diagnosed on a subsequent admission. Caro (1993) reports that in several members of a family he has known for 25 years schizophrenia preceded Huntington's chorea. One member is now (in 1993) diagnosed as schizophrenic and is without signs of Huntington's chorea.

1.9.4 Neurosis

Bolt (1970) noted that among 334 subjects with Huntington's chorea 96 were misdiagnosed at first psychiatric admission. Of these 15% (5% of the whole sample) were included in the category 'neurosis and personality disorder'. In 11 Huntington's patients not referred for psychiatric symptoms but who were subjected to extensive psychiatric assessment, Folstein *et al.* (1979) found four with reactive depression among eight who were identified as psychiatrically abnormal by the General Health Questionnaire (Goldberg, 1972) and among 186 choreics Folstein *et al.* (1987) reported 4·8% as dysthymic disorder. Boll *et al.* (1971) used the Minnesota Multiphasic Personality Inventory (MMPI) to screen out emotional disorders in comparing 9 pairs of matched subjects from each of whom one was Huntington's chorea and the other cerebral damage. In both groups the more impaired in motor skills and problem-solving showed most psychopathology. Mean scores and profiles were not different between the two groups.

1.9.5 Alcoholism

Evidence of the prevalence of alcoholism in Huntington's chorea has been reviewed by King (1985), who found in the literature that both excess of alcohol abuse and a prevalence no greater than that of the general population have each been reported by several authors. To resolve the question he ascertained the prevalence of alcoholism in 45 randomly selected subjects with Huntington's chorea from the pedigrees of the representative sample of the Maryland Survey of Huntington's chorea (Folstein *et al.* 1987). The overall prevalence was 17% (males 24%, females 6%). This prevalence is similar to the lifetime alcohol abuse/dependence found in the general population by Robins *et al.* (1984) to be 25% for males, 4% for females and 14% overall for Baltimore. He concluded that Huntington's chorea does not increase the risk of alcoholism. In this most thorough study of alcoholism in Huntington's chorea to date this result seems conclusive and we have not included alcoholism in our investigation.

1.9.6 Behaviour disorder

In a paper entitled 'Personality Disorder in Huntington's Disease' (1970) Dewhurst reports that among 69 cases of Huntington's chorea from a single kindred of six generations, 20% were categorized as personality disorder at the onset of Huntington's chorea. Ten were admitted to a psychiatric hospital before development of chorea and there diagnosed as personality disorder and several others had been repeatedly convicted. In many cases on follow-up the disordered behaviour continued until it was obscured or submerged by dementia, or the patient died. Two subjects from the same kindred, however, unaffected with chorea but with severe behaviour disorder were followed up long enough to show that they achieved a settled life, married and showed no disturbed behaviour thereafter. Furthermore, three half-siblings from the same mother unaffected with Huntington's chorea and a different unaffected father also developed severe personality disorders. Dewhurst points out that earlier accounts (Hughes, 1925; Rosenbaum, 1941; Chandler *et al.* 1960; Brothers, 1964) reported a high incidence of disturbance of temperament and behaviour, particularly in the prodromal phase of Huntington's chorea. Arguing from his own cases, Dewhurst suggested 'that adverse environmental factors rather than a deleterious gene are likely to cause a behaviour disorder'. The weights to be assigned to each of these factors in the cases at 50% initial risk for Huntington's chorea cannot be determined from the clinical findings however, and it seems equally possible that behaviour disorders can be attributed either to environmental (exogenous) or genetic (endogenous) influences or to their combined influence.

In a historical outline of this dilemma in psychiatry, Lewis (1971) has traced its extensive roots. The difficulty, as he points out, is that 'the external causes which justified the term "exogenous" [are] manifest, identifiable, and even measurable; the internal causes of "endogenous" disorders [are] hypothetical, intangible, elusive predispositions, constitutional or hereditary forces which could be conjectured but not demonstrated'. In the case in point, the relative influence of the Huntington gene in the production of behaviour disorders cannot be determined although in the future it is conceivable that the pathology of gene action may give this information. Personality disorders must be classified by the type of behaviour or change of temperament displayed.

1.9.7 Personality disorder

In the course of Huntington's chorea change of temperament and attitude may occur in the absence of disorder classifiable as psychotic or neurotic. These are alterations in the premorbidly stable characteristics of an affected subject manifesting as morbid jealousy, suspicion, irritability, aggression, stubbornness, egocentricity, apathy, negligence, indifference to responsibility and social obligations, self-neglect or lack of control and restraint, or the like. They are excessive individually in that they are more easily provoked, more frequent, and more disproportionate to the precipitating stimulus than had previously been characteristic. These changes vary in prominence according to the circumstances in which they are reported or ascertained. Irritability and aggression, for instance, are more likely in our experience to come to notice and to be disclosed by a relative in a domestic than in an out-patient setting.

Using DSM-III categories, 5·9% of the 186 cases on the Maryland survey showed antisocial personality (Folstein *et al.* 1987). A problem arises here in categorizing psychiatric disorder associated with Huntington's chorea. Both ICD-9 (WHO, 1978) and DSM-III (APA, 1980) in defining their criteria emphasize that manifestation of personality disorder occur by adolescence or earlier. To qualify as being associated with Huntington's chorea, however, it is necessary that, except for the rare juvenile onset, a change in attitudes, reactions and conduct should have occurred after the time at which personality can be assumed to have developed fully and stabilized. In the study of Folstein (1987) quoted above there is an implication that this is the case, but it is not explicitly stated, and the DSM-III category 'intermittent explosive disorder' is exclusively employed.

It can be seen that behaviour disorder provides the evidence on which temperamental or personality disorder is based. In the present study both aspects are included in the term 'Personality and Behaviour Disorder'.

1.9.8 Irritability

Irritability is among the most frequently found of psychiatric symptoms. Among 150 cases found in an Australian survey, the most frequent psychiatric disturbance was irritability and quick temper found in 70% of cases where mental symptoms preceded chorea (Brothers & Meadows, 1955). In a Scottish population survey of 3 million, which yielded 334 records of Huntington's chorea at all stages, Bolt (1970) noted irritability and violence (50%) as the most frequently recorded clinical feature. Among 30 cases of Huntington's chorea intensively examined by Caine & Shoulson (1983) and categorized by DSM-III (1980) criteria, two cases (7%) showed intermittent explosive disorder. Thirty-one per cent in this category were found at some time during the course of their illness in the 186 cases of the Huntington disease survey of Maryland (Folstein *et al.* 1987).

Ratings on scales of irritability, aggression and apathy were made by Burns and colleagues (1990) from interviews with relatives on 26 subjects with Huntington's chorea and 31 with Alzheimer's disease randomly selected from outpatients and a comparison group of unaffected relatives. The two affected groups showed the same proportion (58%) who were irritable, but aggression was significantly more marked in Huntington's than in Alzheimer's subjects. It was also more frequently rated ($P < 0.01$), more severe (NS) and lasted longer ($P < 0.005$). In both groups aggressive outbursts were precipitated by a preceding event such as an argument between spouses about money. In both Huntington's and Alzheimer's subjects ratings of aggression were greatly in excess of those of the controls. Irritability was correlated with the premorbid trait 'bad tempered' ($P < 0.01$) but was not associated with pre-morbid aggression.

From an examination of 32 hospital case records, Tamir *et al.* (1969) found significantly more male than female patients with Huntington's chorea were aggressive.

1.10 THE RELATION BETWEEN HUNTINGTON'S CHOREA AND FUNCTIONAL PSYCHIATRIC DISORDER

The diagnosis of Huntington's chorea can be made correctly by experienced psychiatrists with thorough investigation in practically all cases, except for the 3% with onset at 60 years or over, where a proportion are handicapped by concurrent illness and failure to yield family history (Folstein *et al.* 1986) is more frequent. The duration from onset to death has been found by Conneally (1984) to be independent of age of onset and remarkably constant, with a mean of 17 years and a range of 14 to 18 years (except for the 2% with onset below 10 or exceeding 69 years, where the mean is 9). A likely influence on the frequency of onset of functional psychiatric disorder is therefore the period during the course of Huntington's chorea at which this occurs. This can conveniently be measured by the time between the onset of functional psychiatric disorder and the onset of chorea.

We may note from the survey of previous studies that in the diagnosis of functional psychiatric disorder in Huntington's chorea problems over diagnosis remain. This relates especially to schizophrenia and to behaviour and personality disorder. Standardized psychiatric methods do not satisfactorily match symptomatology relating to these two disorders as it is encountered in Huntington's chorea.

1.11 AIMS OF THE STUDY

1. Our first purpose was to obtain a representative sample of subjects affected with Huntington's chorea with demographic features measured and to estimate the adult frequency of first onset of functional psychiatric disorder. (N.B. 'Psychiatric disorder' comprises psychiatric illness and personality and behaviour disorder. In this study the term 'psychiatric illness' does not include personality and behaviour disorder.)

2. To examine the distribution of the first onset of functional psychiatric disorder in time over the course of Huntington's chorea.

3. To compare the frequency of functional psychiatric disorder in asymptomatic subjects at 50% initial risk for Huntington's chorea with that of their cohabiting spouses.

4. To examine the effect of the Huntington's gene on the onset of functional psychiatric disorder in subjects at 50% initial risk by comparison of onset of these disorders with that of their non-gene-carrying spouses.

5. To estimate the effect of the Huntington's chorea gene on the first onset of functional psychiatric disorders by comparing its frequency in gene carriers and non-choreic gene carriers as revealed by the predictive genetic linkage test.

Method

2.1 SOURCE OF DATA

2.1.1 The Oxford Regional Health Authority

The Department of Medical Genetics, located in the Churchill Hospital, Oxford, provides a service for the four counties (population 2·52 million) forming the administrative area of the Oxford Regional Health Authority under the National Health Service (Fig. 1). Out-patient clinics provide genetic consultant services in all the NHS general hospitals which together cover the Region, to which general practitioners and consultants in other specialties refer cases. Kindred or family members living outside the Oxford Region may be served by other regional departments, according to where they reside, which, for genetic investigations, will require exchange of information between consultants of different Regions. It is sometimes convenient to agree that one Region should deal with families divided between two or more Regions. Not all Regional Genetic Departments have the resources in staff and experience to maintain a DNA laboratory capable of carrying out pre-symptomatic linkage analyses in Huntington's chorea and patients will then be referred to the most conveniently situated department of a neighbouring Region. The Oxford Regional Department of Medical Genetics had assembled resources and gained considerable expertise in linkage analysis for some years before the advent of a presymptomatic linkage test in Huntington's chorea.

2.1.2 Subjects

Our subjects were the affected and unaffected members of families with Huntington's chorea who were interested in the presymptomatic linkage test for the gene for Huntington's chorea and living within Oxford Regional Health Authority. In 1985–6 a letter was sent to all families who had previously been referred to and seen by the Medical Genetics Department of the Churchill Hospital, Oxford, for Hunting-ton's chorea, offering an interview to explain the test. To this number was added new referrals for Huntington's chorea from 1985 to 1990.

Families of subjects referred to the Department of Medical Genetics were interviewed either in their homes or at hospital out-patient departments by a psychiatrist and a community nursing sister attached to the department. After the diagnosis of Huntington's chorea had been established, the interview had several purposes: (1) to give information about Huntington's chorea and its mode of transmission, and to explain the linkage test and what it entails; (2) to examine affected individuals and take a clinical history; (3) to obtain a history of psychiatric disorder from individuals; (4) to take 20 ml of blood from family members as a source of each individual's DNA for the linkage test; (5) to locate other affected family members; (6) to assemble pedigrees of affected kindreds; and (7) to initiate counselling for individuals.

2.1.3 Assessments for establishing the diagnosis of Huntington's chorea in families

The requirements for diagnosis of Huntington's chorea are the presence of movement disorder, with dementia and a family history showing a dominant mode of transmission. A post-mortem examination is the most useful additional in-formation as it gives unequivocal evidence of Huntington's chorea. A certain diagnosis is mandatory for a family undergoing linkage testing as an error would mean that the test results given to subjects in that family would be wrong: subjects would be told either that they had or had not a high risk of developing Huntington's chorea, or that their children either had 50% or had no chance of receiving the Huntington's gene from them. In fact, there would either be no risk or, if another dominant disorder was present, all offspring of the subject would present an initial 50% risk of inheriting it.

In developed cases of Huntington's chorea, when chorea and dementia are present and affected parents, sibs or children can be ex-amined, diagnosis offers little difficulty. Both

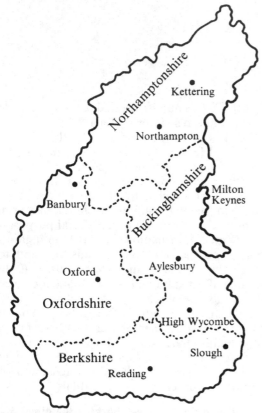

FIG. 1. Oxford Region 1988. Showing the counties and towns that have genetic clinics.

dementia and chorea, however, have an insidious onset, so that at an early stage diagnosis may have to await progress of the disease. In obtaining a family history affected relatives may not be available for examination through death, distance or unwillingness, and the diagnosis will then depend on hospital reports. This will be most valuable and reliable when there is a report of a post mortem examination on the brain, which, however, is uncommon.

It is important to establish whether there are enough family members available who are suitable and willing to enable information from a presymptomatic linkage analysis test to be obtained for any family members, as is described in section 2.2.

2.1.4 Types of subject

For our purpose the subjects fell into three classes: (1) affected, (2) at risk, and (3) spouses. The affected were those in whom a diagnosis of

Huntington's chorea had been or could be made. Those at an initial 50% risk for developing Huntington's chorea were the children or siblings of Huntington's choreics. Subjects at lesser risk (e.g. grandchildren of a Huntington's choreic at 25% initially) are not included in the study. The spouse (or 'married in') of a Huntington's choreic or an at-risk person carried no risk of developing the disease but shared the family environment. Martello *et al.* (1978) point out that although on average 50% of the offspring of a parent affected with Huntington's chorea will carry the Huntington's gene and thus all offspring will bear at birth a 50% risk of developing the disease, should they live long enough, the risk for any individual varies according to age and the period for which the risk is calculated. This is because: (1) some individuals may die before reaching the age of manifestation; (2) as the disease manifests itself the proportion of heterozygotes among non-affected offspring decreases; and (3) the probability of manifestation within a given age interval increases as the individual approaches the age of most frequent manifestation and decreases as it is passed. These authors supply instructions for making corrections in the light of these considerations which must be applied in counselling individuals and in making relevant epidemiological calculations. These circumstances do not apply here, however, and we will continue for convenience to refer to our groups of first-degree blood-relatives of affected subjects as asymptomatic subjects at an initial 50% risk.

2.1.5 A representative sample of affected subjects

A sample was drawn of all subjects with Huntington's chorea and residing within the catchment area of the Oxford Regional Health Authority (Fig. 1) in 1988 in the following way. Subjects from affected families who were referred to the Medical Genetics Department up to the end of 1988 were visited and were examined by members of the research team. Those who were affected, alive and resident during 1988 in any of the four counties comprising the Oxford Region were selected and a psychiatric history was completed for inclusion in the representative sample, of which they formed section C (Fig. 2). To these were added those who were referred subsequently to 1988 from whom subjects who

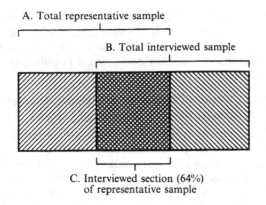

A. Total representative sample

B. Total interviewed sample

C. Interviewed section (64%)
of representative sample

A. All affected subjects, alive and resident in Oxford
Region, 1988 ($N = 101$)

B. All affected subjects for whom psychiatric history
was obtained ($N = 101$)

C. All affected subjects alive and resident in Oxford
region 1988 for whom psychiatric history was
obtained ($N = 65$)

FIG. 2. Composition of samples of subjects in the Oxford Regional
Health Authority affected with Huntington's chorea.

were affected and living in the Oxford Region in
1988 were selected. These latter selections however were not interviewed psychiatrically and
information regarding the history of functional
psychiatric disorder was not obtained. The total
representative sample (A, Fig. 2) therefore
consisted of subjects referred to the Medical
Genetics Department to the end of 1988 together
with subjects subsequently referred but not
psychiatrically interviewed who were affected
and alive in 1988.

A pedigree was drawn of each family of
subjects referred to the genetic department, to
elucidate the pattern of inheritance displayed by
the illness for diagnosis and to estimate the risk
of contracting the disease for unaffected members and their descendants. This assisted in
compiling a complete relevant family history.

2.1.6 Total interviewed sample of affected subjects

As well as the representative samples, a total
interviewed sample (B, Fig. 2) was formed of all
the subjects who were psychiatrically examined
(101) irrespective of whether they fulfilled the
residential condition for inclusion in the representative sample. The reason for this sample
was to provide a required larger number of

affected subjects for a purpose for which a
representative sample was not necessary (see
3.1.6).

2.1.7 Sample of subjects at an initial 50 % risk for Huntington's chorea

First-degree relatives of affected subjects who
display no evidence of Huntington's chorea
form the group of subjects who carry an initial
50 % risk of manifesting the disease at some time
in their lives. The label 'initial 50 % risk' is
convenient for distinguishing these members of
Huntington's families from subjects who are
affected. It must be borne in mind, however, that
different individual values can be given to the
risk according, for instance, to age or whether
the result of presymptomatic linkage test has
been ascertained. Irrespective of these considerations, the label 'initial 50 % risk' indicates for
our purposes simply that the subject is an
unaffected first-degree blood relative of a person
diagnosed as being affected with Huntington's
chorea.

2.1.8 Controls for subjects at initial 50 % risk

For the purpose of distinguishing the separate
effects of gene and environment on the production of functional psychiatric disorder the
cohabiting spouses of subjects at initial 50 %
risk were used as controls. They were assumed
to be at zero risk of carrying the Huntington's
gene but shared the family environment with
their marriage partner.

2.1.9 The prevalence of Huntington's chorea and the completeness of samples

Our estimate of the prevalence of Huntington's
chorea is calculated from the number of affected
subjects living in the Oxford Health Region
during 1988 (A, Fig. 2) as a proportion of its
general population. For this purpose the com-
pleteness of referrals to the Medical Genetics
Department is mandatory and referral is de-
pendent upon medical and public knowledge of
the presymptomatic linkage test. In principle the
test became available in 1983 but a probe was
not made available to the Oxford department
until 1985 and even then there was a delay in
procuring the resources, facilities and agreements
necessary for proceeding with the test. In the
meantime, however, knowledge concerning the
procedure was disseminated through contact

with Huntington's families previously referred and considerable medical and lay publicity was given to its availability. The value of the test was principally to young adults at initial 50% risk and their prospective or actual marriage partners who were given a considerably improved opportunity of learning about the disease and the test. The necessity of including the largest possible number of family members, affected and unaffected, in the test reinforced the confidence of these referends in imparting a complete family history and of older family members in using access to expert knowledge of the disease. General practitioners, neurologists and psychiatrists also saw in their knowledge of the test a more compelling purpose for referring subjects.

The nearest alternative sites to Oxford for referral were London, Birmingham and Cardiff. A small number of Oxford Regional residents had contacts with these and other centres because some part of their family had been living and referred there. Such cases, however, were usually finally dealt with in the Oxford Region for their own convenience and information was obtained on the few who were not. By 1990 it seems most likely that all persons affected up to 1988 were ascertained and referred as the interests of Huntington's families had been converted to referral to a Genetics Department and to full confidential disclosure of the individual and family histories by the advent of the widely publicized test.

Although the whole history of functional psychiatric disorder in individual patients was examined for making a diagnosis only one attack of each illness or disorder, the first, along with its date of onset, was counted for each subject.

2.1.10 The frequency of functional psychiatric disorder in Huntington's chorea

The frequency of functional psychiatric disorder (including illness, personality and behaviour disorder) in Huntington's chorea is the number of cases disclosing a history of the disorder on psychiatric examination, among all cases of Huntington's chorea living in the Oxford Region in 1988. Only 67% of the cases had a psychiatric examination, however, and it is from these (C, Fig. 2) that the prevalence of functional psychiatric disorder is derived. The representative

sample of affected persons (A, Fig. 2) and the 67% samples (C, Fig. 2) were compared for age to test their homogeneity and thus whether the assumption that they are a single population is justified.

2.1.11 Onset of functional psychiatric disorder in relation to onset of Huntington's chorea

The time of onset or of professional recognition of functional psychiatric disorder occurring in Huntington's chorea is noted in a number of studies (see Introduction) as preceding the onset of Huntington's chorea or occurring at various stages in the course of the patient's hospitalization. Folstein (1989, p. 139) divides the 15 to 19-year course of Huntington's chorea into three approximately 5-year stages with the type and amount of care required mainly in mind. She mentions, some clinical observations however; that the majority of depressive attacks occur by the completion of the first stage and the difference in the progress of dementia between Huntington's and Alzheimer's Disease by Stage 3. The relation of the onset of functional psychiatric disorders in relation to the onset of Huntington's chorea has not previously been studied systematically, however, and we have undertaken this in the present study.

In subjects interviewed by the research team the years of onset of functional psychiatric disorder and of Huntington's chorea were obtained. The onset of Huntington's chorea and the periods adjacent to it were divided into three stages (Fig. 13): (1) before onset; (2) during onset; and (3) after onset. The onset of functional psychiatric disorder was allocated to one of these stages. For subjects in whom more than one category of functional psychiatric disorder was diagnosed, the onsets of all syndromes were separately included.

2.1.12 The ascertainment of functional psychiatric disorder in Huntington's chorea

The psychiatric history was directed to obtaining a description of the symptoms and changes of behaviour which had occurred and dating their onset to a year. Initially, the Present State Examination (Wing *et al.* 1974) was administered to subjects who had a positive psychiatric history. This was abandoned, however, as subjects rarely displayed psychiatric disturbance beyond distress, worry or apprehension at the time of interview, or subjects were sometimes too demented to allow examination. The frequency of symptoms, syndromes and changed behaviours was therefore assessed from the clinical history obtained.

The most obvious psychiatric disorder occurring in Huntington's chorea is dementia. The term 'functional psychiatric disorder' is employed here however to refer to other psychiatric disorders, for which brain pathology or disease has not been demonstrated as a cause and, as they occur *per se* do not show the cognitive deterioration of dementia. Functional psychiatric disorder in Huntington's chorea is classified according to general psychiatric practice and separated on the one hand into manifestations which resemble common psychiatric illnesses and on the other into personality and behaviour disorders.

The clinical pictures found in Huntington's chorea which resemble, and are indistinguishable from, functional psychiatric illness have been described by Folstein (1989) as predominantly affective disorder and schizophrenia from the ascertainment of all subjects in whom symptoms and syndromes had occurred up to the time of survey (1980–3) and who were affected with

Huntington's chorea and alive in the state of Maryland (population 4·2 million) on 1 April 1980. In attempting to apply standardized diagnostic criteria to affected subjects to ascertain these disorders, we frequently found that although suggestive symptoms were included in the history or elicited at interview, the clinical picture appeared fragmentary on examination and when dementia had advanced only vestiges remained. The use of a standardized diagnostic schedule was therefore inappropriate. Instead, during interviews, subjects and/or relatives were asked whether they had at any time suffered from nervous or psychiatric illness, or a change in personality and behaviour, and enquiries were made about medical consultations, medications and time off work. A clinical history was taken if an affirmative response to these questions was received. The interview covered illness behaviour included in the items shown in Table 3.

A diagnosis was made under one of the following categories: (1) minor depression; (2) major depression; (3) schizophrenia; (4) personality and behaviour disorder; (5) other functional psychiatric illness; and (6) no functional psychiatric disorder.

Depression

Depressive disorder was divided into major and minor categories. Table 4 shows the categories included from the International Classification of Diseases (ICD-9) and DSM-III. Depression manifesting at least two of the features shown in Table 5 was taken to be minor depression.

Table 3. *Items of illness behaviour included in diagnostic interview of HC family members*

1 General practitioner consultation
2 Referral to psychiatrist
3 Medication prescribed: how long?
4 Duration of illness
5 Absence from work: how long?
6 Precipitant of illness

Table 4. *Categories included in classification of depression, schizophrenia and personality disorder occurring in association with Huntington's chorea*

Depression	Minor depression	Major depression
ICD-9 (1978)	309.0 Brief depressive reaction	296 Affective psychosis
	300.4 Neurotic depression	
DSM-III (1980)	309.0 Adjustment disorder	296.2, 296.3 Major depression
	– depressed mood	300.4 Dysthymic disorder
Schizophrenia		
ICD-9	295, 297 Schizophrenic and paranoid disorders	
DSM-III	295 Schizophrenia	
Syndrome Check List	Residual syndrome, auditory hallucinations, delusions of persecution, delusions of reference	
Personality and behaviour disorder	Items from published studies shown in Table 3.	

Table 5. *Features of minor depression*

1	Duration less than 7 days
2	Medication less than a month
3	Absence from work less than 7 days
4	A precipitant preceding
5	Anxiety prominent
6	Psychiatric referral

Schizophrenia

For a diagnosis of schizophrenia all material gathered relevant to a diagnosis (history, medical notes, medical letters) were submitted to the Syndrome Check List (Wing *et al.* 1974). Those who met the criteria for nuclear or residual syndromes, auditory hallucinations, delusions of persecution or delusions of reference were diagnosed as schizophrenia. The ICD-9 (WHO, 1978) was the standard used for other functional psychiatric illness.

Personality and behaviour disorder

Both ICD-9 (WHO, 1978) and DSM-III (APA, 1983) conceptualize personality disorder as faulty or deviant *development* of personality traits, generally recognizable by adolescence, which produces inflexible, maladaptive adjustment to other people and in provocative situations. What is encountered in Huntington's chorea, however, is *change* in developed behaviour and temperament occurring most often in mature adults which, compared to what is envisaged in ICD-9 and DSM-III, proceeds more rapidly and is relatively unstable, altering as the brain disorder progresses. The change is more in the form of erosion and disorganization of settled dispositions and disinhibition than faulty development and is referred to in this study as personality and behaviour disorder.

In order to measure the frequency of this condition, therefore, a list of the items of

Table 6. *Items of disordered personality and behaviour occurring in Huntington's chorea extracted from published studies*

Irritable	Jealous
Temper	Quarrelsome
Excitable	Callous
Aggressive	Unrestrained sexually
Impatient	Apathy, neglect
Suspicious	Anxiety

personality and behaviour disorder was compiled from the literature dealing with this topic (Table 6) (Wallace, 1962; Bolt, 1970; Dewhurst *et al.* 1970; Oliver, 1970; Caine & Shoulson, 1983; Folstein, 1989; Pflanz *et al.* 1991) and noted in the clinical history when reported in interview with patient and/or relative.

2.1.13 Effect of environment on production of functional psychiatric illness and disorder in subjects at initial 50% risk

Persons at initial 50% risk of developing Huntington's chorea are those who showed no evidence of the disease but had an affected parent from whom either a normal or mutant Huntington's chorea gene had been transmitted. There is no practical presymptomatic method of detecting the presence of the Huntington's gene until the disease manifests itself except for the linkage test. The onset of functional psychiatric disorder is described by Dewhurst and colleagues (1969) as occurring up to a decade before chorea and being indistinguishable from that occurring unassociated with Huntington's chorea. The occurrence of this disorder may therefore either be coincidental, associated with the family trauma accompanying Huntington's chorea or associated with the presence of the Huntington's chorea gene. To distinguish these alternatives we compared the frequency of psychiatric disorder in subjects at initial 50% risk with that of their cohabiting spouse (at zero risk). Controls could not be found for those unmarried, widowed or separated since blood relatives were either affected or at risk. Stable cohabitees were accepted if the relationship had lasted more than 2 years. In the majority of cases spouses accompanied subjects to the interview, or were seen at home with them. A few spouses were not seen and the information was obtained from the subject or another relative. The history was obtained and a psychiatric diagnosis made as for subjects at initial 50% risk.

Significant evidence for the Huntington's chorea gene as a cause would be provided if functional psychiatric disorder was found at a frequency approaching 50% in subjects at an initial 50% risk for carrying the gene or at a frequency significantly greater than in subjects at zero risk. On the other hand, a frequency of functional psychiatric disorder in subjects at zero risk either approaching equality with or exceeding that in those at initial 50% risk would be evidence in support of an environmental cause of the functional psychiatric disorder.

2.1.14 Effect of Huntington's chorea gene on production of functional psychiatric disorder

Subjects whose presymptomatic linkage test result indicated a high probability of carrying the Huntington's gene were compared in respect of the frequency of a history of functional psychiatric disorder with those where a low probability was indicated. The linkage test results were withheld from research team members until the diagnosis of functional psychiatric disorder and of the types of disorder was made so that clinicians remained blind to the test results and thus ensured that this knowledge did not bias the allocation of the diagnosis of functional psychiatric disorder. A significantly higher frequency of functional psychiatric disorder in the high risk group would indicate influence of the Huntington's gene in its production.

2.1.15 The manifestation of functional psychiatric disorder in other illness than Huntington's chorea

There are a considerable number of studies of functional psychiatric disorder, mainly depression, in the general population, in other types of dementia than that of Huntington's chorea. These have been expressed uniformly as a percentage frequency of the psychiatric condition to allow comparison with the percentage frequency we have found for Huntington's chorea.

2.2 THE GENETIC BASIS OF THE TEST FOR ESTIMATING THE PROBABILITY OF DEVELOPING HUNTINGTON'S CHOREA IN SUBJECTS AT INITIAL 50% RISK

The predictive test utilizes the techniques of molecular biology to track the inheritance of the Huntington's chorea (HC) gene using linked DNA markers in families with the disease, thus enabling predictions of the status of asymptomatic but at risk relatives to be made. The following sections outline the principles and methodology applied in this study. It is not intended to be a complete overview of the application of molecular genetics but for the benefit of those readers unfamiliar with the molecular basis of inheritance a brief introduction has been included. For further details and information about this rapidly expanding field the reader is referred to the following textbooks (Davies & Read, 1988; Strachan, 1992).

2.2.1 The molecular basis of inheritance

Nucleic acids

Nucleic acids are the molecules which carry genetic information in man as well as other organisms. Their function is to direct protein synthesis and transmit all this information accurately from one generation to the next. There are two types of nucleic acid, DNA (deoxyribonucleic acid) and RNA (ribonucleic acid) each composed of long chains of nucleotides. Each nucleotide consist of three moieties – (1) sugar (deoxyribose in DNA, ribose in RNA); (2) phosphate; and (3) nitrogenous bases. In DNA there are 4 nitrogenous bases, two purines – adenine (A) and guanine (G) – and two pyrimidines – cytosine (C) and thymine (T). The nitrogenous bases found in RNA differ in one respect only, that is thymine is replaced by uracil (U) (Fig. 3).

Structure of DNA

DNA is made up of two nucleotide chains wound round each other in the form of a double helix. The backbone of the chain is made up of the sugar–phosphate moieties of each nucleotide while the nitrogenous bases project into the double helix where they form hydrogen bonds with the bases of the other strand. Hydrogen (H) bonds can only be formed between A and T and C and G. Thus, the overall appearance of the double helix is that of a flexible ladder twisted on its axis with the H bonded base pairs forming the rungs (Fig. 4). The two strands of DNA which run in opposite orientation are said to be complementary, since the sequence of bases on one strand automatically determines the sequence on the other strand because of the specific pairing of the bases. Therefore if the sequence on one strand is

$$5'\text{-ATGCCAC-}3'$$

the other must be

$$3'\text{-TACGGTG-}5'$$

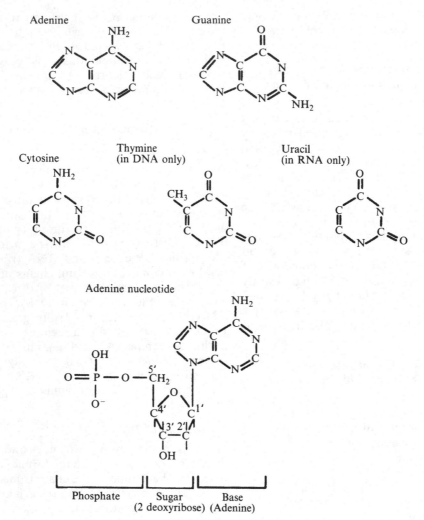

Fig. 3. The individual bases found in DNA and RNA are shown in the top half of the diagram. Note that thymine is replaced by uracil in RNA. A nucleotide consists of a phosphate group attached to the 5′ carbon of the sugar together with a base attached to the 1′ carbon of the sugar. In DNA the sugar is 2-deoxyribose, whereas in RNA it is ribose. The adenine nucleotide found in DNA is shown for example.

Replication of DNA

During replication the two strands of DNA in the double helix unwind at several points along the chromosome. Each strand then acts as a template for the synthesis of new DNA using the enzyme DNA polymerase (Fig. 5). This process of replication is called semi-conservative because only one strand of the resultant daughter molecule is newly synthesized.

Function of nucleic acids

The human genome contains approximately 6×10^9 base pairs (bp) of DNA organized into discrete units called chromosomes. Each diploid cell contains 46 chromosomes, 22 pairs of autosomes and two sex chromosomes, either two X chromosomes in the female or one X and one Y in the male. The gametes are haploid and contain one of each pair of autosomes and one of the two sex chromosomes.

DNA encodes the information required to make protein molecules in units called genes

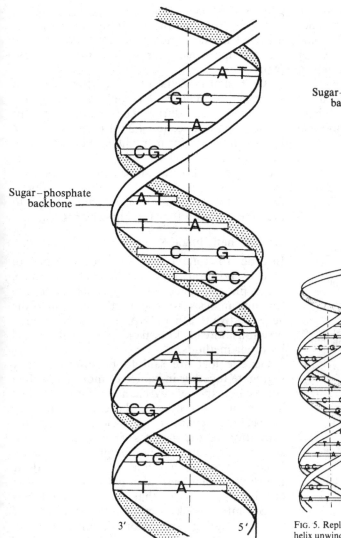

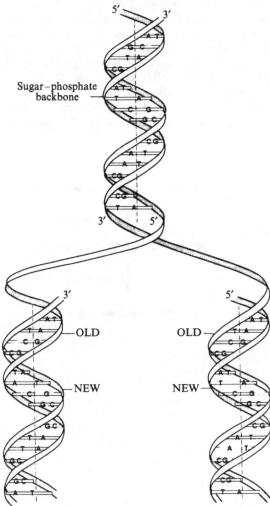

FIG. 4. The structure of DNA. A schematic representation of the double helix showing the specific base pairing of the bases across the helix (i.e. the rungs of the ladder). The backbone of the chain comprises the sugar–phosphate moieties of the nucleotides.

FIG. 5. Replication of DNA. Schematic diagram showing the double helix unwinding to act as a template for the synthesis of two daughter molecules.

with each amino acid in the protein encoded by a specific triplet of nucleotides termed a codon. For example, the triplet CCT encodes the amino acid glycine, whereas GCA codes for arginine. Genes can vary in size from about 2×10^3 base pairs of DNA up to over 2×10^6. For example, the gene coding the protein dystrophin whose disruption leads to Duchenne's muscular dystrophy is 2.3×10^6 base pairs. A gene is composed of 'introns' (non-coding regions) and 'exons' (coding regions). The amount of DNA in the human genome is far in excess of that required to code for the 50–100000 functional genes predicted to be present in man. A proportion of the remainder consists of repetitive DNA, which does not code, and DNA coding for ribosomal and transfer RNAs. Most of the DNA in the mammalian genome is apparently redundant without a clearly defined function.

The process of making protein from DNA requires an intermediary. DNA is transcribed into single stranded messenger RNA (mRNA) in the nucleus, its sequence being complementary to that of the transcribed strand of DNA. The mRNA is then processed to remove the introns and moves into the cytoplasm where it becomes attached to the ribosomes. As the ribosome moves along the mRNA in the process of translation each codon is recognized by a matching transfer (tRNA) molecule. The specific complementary anticodon which adds an amino acid to the growing part of the protein chain finally produces a complete protein molecule (Fig. 6).

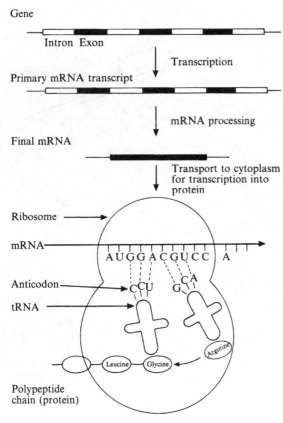

FIG. 6. Transcription of DNA to mRNA and subsequent translation to protein.

Gene regulation

Since all cells of an organism contain the same genetic information there must be a mechanism for controlling gene expression enabling tissues to differentiate and to synthesize different proteins. Apart from initiation and termination codons other regulatory sequences are found both 'upstream' and 'downstream' of a gene

(Fig. 6). The gene promoter is generally found 100 bp upstream of the initiation codon and it is involved in the bonding of RNA polymerase, the enzyme which synthesizes mRNA from DNA.

After many years of effort the gene for Huntington's chorea has only recently been isolated – in fact, during the preparation of this monograph (see section 4.2 for discussion). The approaches used for mapping and closing in on the gene yielded DNA markers linked to the Huntington's chorea gene which could be used for predictive testing. The following sections describe the application of genetic linkage to predictive testing for Huntington's chorea.

2.2.2 Genetic linkage

In order to clone a gene it is necessary first to map its position on a particular chromosome, i.e. define its locus. One approach is to use 'linkage analysis' to establish the position of the gene relative to other DNA markers whose map position is already known or could be determined by other methods.

Genetic loci are said to be linked if they segregate together in pedigrees more often than would be expected by chance. The closer two loci are on a chromosome, the less likely are they to become separated at meiosis during the formation of the gametes when each chromosome pairs with its homologue and recombination or crossing over at specific points along the chromosome pair takes place. The situation can be compared to that in which a joker is placed into a pack of cards of known order of the surrounding cards before shuffling the pack. If the cards are cut and the order then examined one would expect to observe that those cards closest to the joker remain in those relative positions whereas cards further away would most likely have changed order. Genetic distance between two loci is usually measured in units called centimorgans (cM), a unit based on the observed rate of recombination between two loci. As each gamete has about 3×10^9 bp and, on average, has about 30 recombinant events in male meiosis and rather more in the female, each million base pair (a megabase) has a chance of about 1 % if recombining. On average, therefore, a megabase is equivalent to one centimorgan (1 cM). However, this relationship may vary from one chromosomal region to the next due to

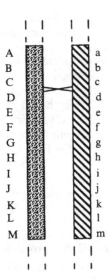

Following a single recombination event, in this case between loci C and D, the chromosomes passed on to the gametes and hence offspring would look like this:

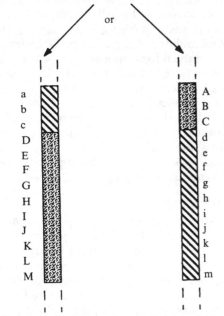

FIG. 7. An example of the use of marker loci to track inheritance.

the presence of recombination 'hotspots' and it also varies between male and female gametes.

The following example of linkage illustrates how marker loci can be used to track the inheritance of a disease locus such as the gene for Huntington's chorea. If the loci on a pair of homologous chromosomes were represented by

the letters A to M, the appearance of the parental pair would be as shown in Fig. 7.

It can be seen that adjacent loci such as E and F are more likely to remain together following meiosis rather than more distant loci such as B and L. Thus, the closer two loci are on a chromosome the more 'tightly linked' they are and the smaller the observed rate of recombination (σ) between them. Loci are said to be tightly linked if the rate of recombination between them is 5% or less. If one observes such tight linkage between a disease locus, whose inheritance can be followed through affected families, and a marker locus, predictions can then be made on the clinical status of the various family members. This is the basis of the predictive test for Huntington's chorea as shown in the following example.

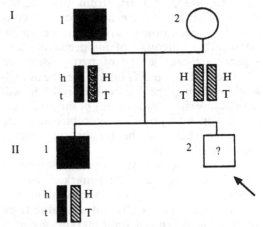

FIG. 8. The basis of the predictive test for Huntington's chorea using a closely linked marker with two alleles (T, t). The disease-causing allele is represented by h and the normal allele by H. → denotes the consultand.

Fig. 8 shows a pedigree in which an asymptomatic individual (II,2) wishes to know whether he will develop the disease in later life. His father is affected and he already has one older sib who has been diagnosed as having the disease. DNA from all members of the pedigree is available. If the gene for Huntington's chorea is represented by h and that for the normal or 'wildtype' allele is represented by H, then all the affected individuals would have the genotype Hh and all normal individuals HH. As has already been stated, we have no direct means of distinguishing alleles H and h because at the time of writing the gene has not been cloned. However, there are

DNA markers available that exist in forms (alleles) which can be distinguished from one another which are tightly linked to the disease gene.

Let such a marker with two alleles be represented by T and t with an observed recombination rate of 5% between the marker and the HC disease locus. Following DNA analysis the individual genotypes for all except the consultand (II, 2) are as shown in the pedigree (Fig. 8). From these results we are able to conclude that Huntington's chorea is probably co-inherited with allele t in this family. This is because the unaffected mother (I, 2) is homozygous for allele T (i.e. has two copies of this allele) and can therefore only pass on T to her offspring. Individual (II, 1) therefore, who is heterozyous for this marker must have received allele t together with HC from his affected father. Although we have not typed the consultand yet we are now in a position to examine some possible outcomes of his predictive test. His genotype can be one of two possibilities either Tt or TT. If he is Tt he will then be at high risk of developing the disease, if he is TT he will then be at low risk. The accuracy of the predictive test will depend upon the recombination rate with the marker and the number of meioses involved (see section 2.2.3).

In practice it is always better to use several linked markers because some markers will be informative for some family members but not others or because DNA is not available from key individuals. When several markers are used it is possible to build up a high or low risk 'haplotype' which can be tracked through the family. Even so, it is not always possible to alter a subject's prior risk, i.e. the test is uninformative.

2.2.3 The accuracy of the predictive test

The results of a linkage test can never be 100% accurate because one must take into account the recombination rate of the marker with the disease gene. In the above case we have already stated that the marker recombines with HC at a rate of 5%. Two meioses are involved in calculating the accuracy of the predictive test for the consultand (II, 2), and the chance that recombination has not occurred in either is 0.95×0.95, or about 90%. The test result is therefore 90% accurate. One can also add into the calculation the age related risk for which

there is published data. However, the key information of the tendency of members of the same family to develop the disease at similar ages is difficult to incorporate and ignored on most computerized solutions.

Other sources of error lie in the certainty of the diagnosis of HC within the family and also the possibility that HC is genetically heterogeneous (i.e. more than one gene at different locations are responsible for HC).

So how does the clinical scientist detect linkage and recombination in practice? The following sections describe genetic markers and their use as DNA probes to track disease genes through pedigrees.

2.2.4 Genetic markers (DNA probes)

Using recombinant DNA techniques, it is possible to clone small pieces of DNA (up to 40 kilobases (kb)) by inserting them into vectors, often plasmids, natural parasites of bacteria, which are capable of replicating independently of the host bacterium (usually strains of *E. coli*). By growing these 'transformed' bacteria, one can obtain millions of copies of the DNA inserts and harvest them for future use as DNA probes. More recently it has become possible to clone very large pieces (up to 2 megabases) of DNA into yeast artificial chromosomes (YACS). If required, these cloned inserts can be mapped to chromosomal locations using various physical techniques and they can also be used as DNA probes to look for genetic linkage to specific disease genes using appropriate pedigrees.

Polymorphisms

(a) *Restriction fragment-length polymorphisms (RFLPs)* For a DNA marker or probe to be of any use in a linkage study it must be capable of detecting alternative forms or alleles at a given locus. Restriction fragment length polymorphisms (RFLPs) are commonly detected when DNA markers are used as probes. Restriction enzymes isolated from bacteria are able to cleave DNA wherever they recognize a specific sequence. The majority of these recognition sequences are between 4 and 8 base pairs long, but this can vary. The shorter the recognition sequence the more frequently one is likely to encounter it in the genome and hence smaller DNA fragments will be produced following digestion with an enzyme recognizing such a sequence. For example, following digestion of human DNA with the restriction enzyme *Eco*R I which recognizes the duplex

GAATTC
CTTAAG

the average expected fragment produced is 3 kb, whereas the average observed fragment produced following digestion with the restriction enzyme *Not* I which recognizes the duplex

GCGGCCGC
CGCCGGCG

is 1000 kb. The majority of recognition sequences are symmetrical in this way and rather inaccurately called palindromes.

Approximately 1 base in 200 varies from one person to the next. The majority of these changes have no functional significance (because the majority of DNA appears to be redundant) and they are inherited stably from one generation to the next. Approximately one in six of these changes results in the creation or abolition of a recognition site for a restriction enzyme, and therefore creates a polymorphism which is stably inherited. For example if two non-variant *Eco*R I restriction sites are located 8 kb apart on DNA from two homologous chromosomes, then following digestion with the enzyme each chromosome will produce an 8 kb restriction fragment. If one of the pair also possesses a polymorphic site as shown (Fig. 9) fragments of 5 kb and 3 kb will be produced from the chromosome with the polymorphic site whereas the other will produce a fragment of 8 kb alone.

If our marker DNA to be used as a probe is derived from this region as shown in the diagram, then it will bind to the 5 kb fragment on chromsome A and the 8 kb fragment on chromosome B, thus detecting an RFLP with two alleles of 5 and 8 kb.

(*b*) *Variable number tandem repeats (VNTRs)*
Another type of polymorphism which can be detected in the genome is called a variable number tandem repeat (VNTR) (Fig. 10). This type of polymorphism is characterized by alleles which vary in size by an integral number of basic repeat units. There are several varieties of VNTRs derived from different types of repeat units. For example, satellite DNA usually found near the centromere of the chromosome consists of tandemly repeated units of the order of 100 kb in size, while minisatellite DNA consists of moderately sized arrays (up to 20 kb long) dispersed throughout the genome and thirdly microsatellite DNA which is made up of simple repeat units usually 1–4 bp in length and includes the family of 'CA' dinucleotide repeats which occur on average every 50 kb and are extremely polymorphic.

VNTRs are detected by making use of restriction enzymes which cut the DNA outside of the region containing the tandem array. The alleles produced are therefore a function of the length of the repeated unit.

The techniques used to visualize RFLPs and

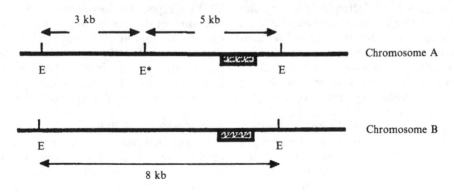

E, *Eco*R I site; E*, polymorphic *Eco*R I site

: Probe

FIG. 9. Diagrammatic representation of a restriction fragment-length polymorphism (RFLP).

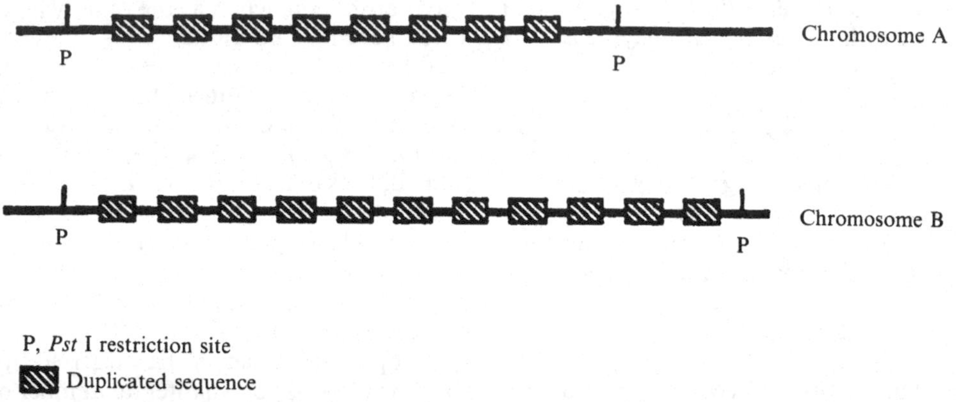

P, *Pst* I restriction site

▧ Duplicated sequence

FIG. 10. Diagrammatic representation of the polymorphisms created by a variable number tandem repeat (VNTR).

VNTRs at the time of publication are described in the following section.

2.2.5 Southern blotting and molecular hybridization

At the first stage in the process of determining whether a piece of cloned DNA will be a useful probe (often called a marker) in a linkage study one must determine whether or not it is capable of detecting an RFLP or VNTR polymorphism. To do this, samples of DNA from a series of unrelated normal individuals are digested with a battery of restriction enzymes (e.g. *Eco*R I, *Hin*d III, *Pst* I, *Taq* I). The digested DNA is then loaded on to agarose gels and sorted according to size by electrophoresis. DNA is negatively charged and therefore will move in the gel towards the positive electrode, the smaller fragments being able to move more quickly than the larger fragments. The distance a fragment will move in the gel following a period of electrophoresis is proportional to the size of the DNA fragment. The DNA is transferred by capillary action following denaturation producing single stranded DNA from the gel to a membrane by the process of Southern blotting. The DNA binds very strongly to the charged membrane and (filter) is now suitable for molecular hybridization with the probe DNA. The probe DNA is first labelled with ^{32}P radioactivity and then denatured. It is then placed in a bag containing a viscous 'hybridization' solution together with the filter and usually left overnight at 65 °C to allow hybridization to occur. The conditions and the composition of the hybridization fluid are such that hybridiza-

tion or annealing of the probe DNA to its complementary DNA sequence on the filter is optimized. Following this period the filter is removed from the bag and washed in a series of solutions with decreasing salt concentration to aid the removal of non-specific binding of the probe DNA to the filter. This is termed stringency washing. The filter is then air dried and autoradiographed (see Fig. 11) to visualize the results. The most useful marker/enzyme combination will be the one for which most individuals are heterozygous, that is bear two distinguishable alleles at a given locus.

Minisatellite VNTRs can also be detected by the above technique. Recently, however, the technique of polymerase chain reaction (PCR) has been adapted to detect many RFLPs and VNTRs, especially the microsatellite CA repeats. Accounts of this powerful technique are given in recent molecular biology textbooks (e.g. Strachan, 1992) and are not described here since the results reported in this study have all been obtained using the techniques of Southern blotting and molecular hybridization.

2.2.6 Establishing linkage

Once a cloned piece of DNA has been shown to detect a polymorphism it can be used in family studies to test for linkage to a particular disease phenotype. The aim is to determine whether within a family a certain allele detected by the marker co-segregates within the disease. It is important in any linkage study that the family structures are suitable. The best pedigrees are those with at least three generations and several affected and non-affected sibs. It was in this way

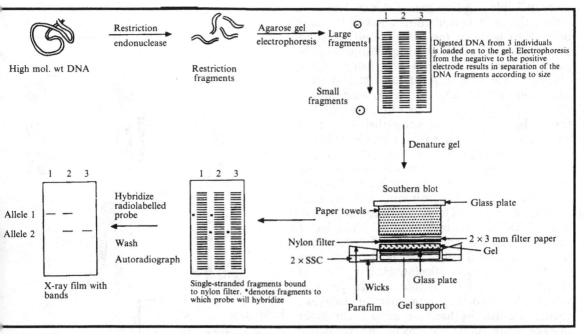

FIG. 11. Southern blotting and molecular hybridization.

that Gusella *et al.* (1983) demonstrated close linkage of the anonymous marker G8 to Huntington's chorea within an enormous Venezuelan HC pedigree, thus allowing the first predictive tests to be undertaken.

2.2.7 The predictive test protocol in the Department of Medical Genetics, Churchill Hospital, Oxford

The subjects at an initial 50% risk who agreed to participate in this study fell into two categories: (*a*) those who did not wish to know the outcome of their results (i.e. had given samples for research only or to assist other family members); and (*b*) those who wished to be informed. It was important that the latter category entered into the approved predictive test counselling programme aimed at preparing the subjects for receipt of their high- or low-risk results. The protocol adopted in this department was derived using guidelines issued by COMBAT (Dalby, 1986) and published protocols from other leading centres (e.g. Fox *et al.* 1989; Crauford & Tyler, 1992).

Most of the families studied contained subjects from both categories, and therefore samples to be analysed for research purposes only were generally processed according to the schedule

for those entering the predictive test programme as outlined below.

Before being accepted on to the predictive test programme, subjects were required to attend 'pre-test counselling sessions' during which the diagnosis of HC within the family was verified as far as possible, accurate family histories and pedigrees were taken, and the nature of the test and the likelihood that DNA analysis would give an informative result (high or low risk) was explained. Additionally, the subjects were given the opportunity to discuss their own particular situation and the implications of the test for themselves, such as effect on their employment, insurance premiums, obtaining a mortgage, and on their personal relationships. These discussions were intended to enable the subject to make an informed decision whether or not to proceed with the test. At this stage blood was collected from all available family members (including those who wished to have the test done for research only) but not from the subject requesting to know the outcome of the predictive test. Following DNA extraction according to published protocols (Sambrook *et al.* 1989), the families were then analysed for 'informativity' by the methods outlined in sections 2.2.2–2.2.5 using the probe/enzyme marker combinations given in Table 7. A time gap of at least 3 months before the next consultation allowed the laboratory to perform the analysis and gave the subjects time to reflect on the implications of the predictive test. The subjects were then given the results of the first stage of the test and were again counselled to help them make an informed decision whether to proceed with the predictive test. Subjects wishing to know their test result who were uninformative at the time were advised that future developments in the field could lead to the isolation of new markers which could make the test informative for them. The department undertook to maintain regular contact with these subjects. Those who were informative and wished to proceed then had their blood taken for analysis and a period of at least one month elapsed before the final result was available. Risks were calculated using published recombination rates combined with pedigree information according to the method of Bayes's theorem, either by hand or using a computer linkage programme (M-link). The predictive tests in this study were carried out over a period of 4 years, during which time closer and more informative markers became available. Therefore, the accuracy of the tests performed in the later stages of this study was likely to be greater than for those undertaken earlier on and this was reflected in the discussion of probability with the patient during counselling. Once the subjects had been informed of their altered risks, regular follow-up was made regardless of the outcome of the test. Fig. 12 shows the results obtained following DNA analysis of one of the families entering the predictive test.

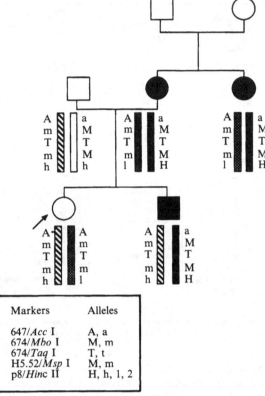

Markers	Alleles
647/*Acc* I	A, a
674/*Mbo* I	M, m
674/*Taq* I	T, t
H5.52/*Msp* I	M, m
p8/*Hinc* II	H, h, 1, 2

FIG. 12. An example of the predictive test carried out in this study. The consultand (→), aged 28 years had a brother, mother and aunt affected by the disease and wished to know her risk of developing HC. Analysis of the DNA from the affected relatives and her father with the markers shown identified the high-risk haplotype (black chromosome) and indicated that the test would be informative with the marker/enzyme combination 674/ *Acc* and p8/ *Hinc* II. Analysis of the consultand's DNA indicated inheritance of the low-risk haplotype from the affected mother. Using the closest informative marker (674) with a recombination fraction of 2% combined with her age-modified risk (penetrance function) it was possible to reduce the consultand's risk at birth of 50% to 3·6%.

Table 7. *Probe/enzyme combinations used for the predictive tests undertaken in this study*

Probe name	Restriction enzyme	Allele size (Kb)	Recombination fraction (%)	Ref.
H5.52	*Msp* I	3·5; 2·8	4	[1]
YNZ32	*Pst* I	2·3–2·8	3	[2]
358	*Pvu* II	1·6; 2·0; 2·8	3	[2]
674	*Acc* I	6·8; 1·5	2	[3]
	Mbo I	1·2; 0·7; 0·5	2	
	Pst I	8·6; 1·7	2	
	Taq I	2·3; 1·8	2	
kp1.65	*Bgl* I	2·0–2·6	2	[2]
252.3	*Pst* I	2·2–2·6	2	[2]
157.9	*Pst* I	1·8–2·1	2	[2]

[1] Bakker *et al.* 1987.
[2] MacDonald *et al.* (1989).
[3] Wasmuth *et al.* (1988).

Chapter 3

Results

3.1 AFFECTED SUBJECTS

3.1.1 Prevalence

By the end of 1988, 34 families who had been in contact with the Oxford Department of Medical Genetics for Huntington's chorea were identified, visited and given a physical and psychiatric examination. A total of 137 affected persons was ascertained. Of these one was excluded on a finding from post mortem examination of an olivo-cerebellar-pontine degeneration. This very rare condition is dominantly inherited, manifests cerebellar movement disorder and may be difficult to distinguish from Huntington's chorea during life (Marsden, 1982; Padberg & Bruyn, 1986). A further case was retained within the sample although a post mortem of the subject's mother who was presumed to be affected with Huntington's chorea revealed that it was Alzheimer's disease. Two other blood relatives in the family, however, had Huntington's chorea. This is similar to an instance quoted by Caro (1993) where Corsellis identified Alzheimer's disease by post mortem examination in a subject from a Huntington's chorea family. Sixty-five subjects met the two conditions necessary for inclusion in our prevalence estimate, namely being alive in 1988 and living within the four counties (Berkshire, Buckinghamshire, Northamptonshire and Oxfordshire) of the Oxford Regional Health Authority (Fig. 1) with a total population of 2·52 million. These formed C (Fig. 2), the interviewed section of the whole representative sample of affected persons alive in 1988. A further 36 affected subjects referred between 1989 and July 1991 who also met the two conditions, but for whom psychiatric information was not obtained, were added to make a total representative sample of 101 subjects (A, Fig. 2). This gave a prevalence of 40 affected persons per million for the 2·52 million general population of the four counties of the Oxford Health Region. This estimate lies within range of 2·5–100 per million for UK populations given in Harper's (1991) review and 15–75 per million estimated by Caro (1972). It is considerably less than the 92 per million recorded

for East Anglia (population 600000) by Caro (1972) but close to that of Reed & Chandler (1958) for Lower Michigan (population 5 million) at 41 per million.

3.1.2 Age

For the whole representative sample (A, Fig. 2) mean age in 1988 was 51·4 year and for the psychiatrically interviewed section of the sample (C, Fig. 2) was 52·0 year (Table 8). The difference

Table 8. *Comparison of psychiatrically interviewed (C, Fig. 2) with total representative sample of subjects affected with HC (A, Fig. 2) in respect of age in 1988*

Age	Male		Female	
	Sect. C (26) (%)	Sect. A (41) (%)	Sect. C (38) (%)	Sect. A (60) (%)
20–29	3	5	—	—
30–39	11	7	13	18
40–49	37	24	26	23
50–59	19	24	34	30
60–69	11	17	18	15
70–79	14	10	8	5
Mean age	51·6	52·7	52·4	51·0
Number age not known	4		1	

between these two means was not significant and there were only slight differences between men and women in the age distribution of illness. This allows us to take C (Fig. 2), the interviewed section, as representative of the whole representative sample.

3.1.3 Age of onset

Table 9 shows age of onset of the total representative sample (A, Fig. 2). There was no material difference between males and females in mean age of onset or in the distribution of age of onset (Table 9). Eighty per cent were aged between 30–59 year. Four subjects had an onset under 20 years (3 male, 1 female) of whom two were siblings.

Table 9. *Age at onset of subjects affected with Huntington's chorea comprising total representative sample (A, Fig. 2)*

Age	Males (N = 44) (%)	Females (N = 57) (%)	Total (N = 101) (%)
< 20	7	2	4
20–29	5	5	5
30–39	25	28	27
40–49	39	35	37
50–59	9	23	17
60–69	11	7	9
> 70	5	0	2
Mean	44·1	44·3	

Table 10. *The number of affected subjects from a representative sample (Fig. 2C) with a history of functional psychiatric illness*

	Male	Female	Total
N	25	40	65
Minor depression	8 (32%)	10 (25%)	18 (28%)
Major depression	4 (16%)	13 (33%)	17 (26%)
Schizophrenia	4 (16%)	4 (10%)	8 (12%)
Total functional psychiatric illness	16 (64%)	27 (68%)	43 (66%)
No history of functional psychiatric illness	9	13	22

3.1.4 Age of death

The age of death was known for 33 affected subjects whose death was reported and dated by the psychiatrically interviewed families (C, Fig. 2). The last year included was 1979 and the earliest death was in 1942. The age at death was unknown in 7 cases. Mean age of death of 33 subjects was 51·9 year with a range of 35–74. There was no material difference between males and females. Forty-one per cent of subjects died aged between 40 and 59; 30% survived to 60. Eight subjects (five men, three women) were reported to have committed suicide of whom two disappeared and were assumed to be suicides. Thus, from 107 subjects eight committed suicide in seven years.

3.1.5 Functional psychiatric illness in affected subjects

The occurrence of first reported episodes of depression and schizophrenic symptoms in Section C (Fig. 2) of the representative sample is shown in Table 10. Two-thirds of the subjects had a history of these conditions which occurred in approximately equal proportions in the sexes, except for a non-significant excess ($\chi^2 = 2·2$, $P > 0·17$) of major depression in females (Table 10).

The prevalence of depression we have found can be compared with that of Robins *et al.* (1984) for the general population (Table 20). They estimated the lifetime prevalence of major depressive disorder in three urban settings and obtained rates ranging from 3·7% to 6·7%

(average 5%), which is five times less than our estimate for Huntington's chorea.

The 12% of subjects showing schizophrenic symptoms (Table 10) considerably exceeds the 0·9% life expectancy of schizophrenia in the general population to age 60 calculated by Shields (1978) from the Camberwell register.

3.1.6 Frequency of items of behaviour and personality disorder in persons affected with Huntington's chorea

Table 11 demonstrates that about half of the same sample (C, Fig. 2) show personality and behaviour disorder. Men, of whom about half undergo these changes, show a non-significant excess over women ($\chi^2 = 1·1$, $P > 0·1$).

Table 11. *The number of affected subjects from a representative sample (Fig. 2C) with a history of change in behaviour and/or personality*

	Male	Female	Total
N	27	38	65
With	13 (48%)	14 (37%)	27 (42%)
Without	13	24	37
Not known	1 (4%)	0	1 (2%)

Aggressiveness and violence directed mainly against spouses and, less often, children and parents, affect the largest proportion of subjects (about 50%) and next are suspicion (29%) and temper (25%). Other items affect less than 20% of subjects while excitability, callousness and anxiety are hardly recorded. There was no disorder of behaviour and personality in 16% of subjects.

The mean number of items per man (1·83) is higher than for women (1·56). In two specific items a notable excess occurs among males; aggressiveness ($+188\%$, $1 > P > 0·05$) and sexual disinhibition ($+14\%$). A higher proportion of women (12%) than men were quarrelsome. No other difference between men and women exceeds 10%.

Table 12 gives evidence of social disorder which reinforces the impression of a strong tendency to male predominance on violence ($+31·0\%$, $P > 0·05$), marital discord ($+20·9\%$), criminal offence ($+12·5\%$).

Table 12. *Social disorder occurring in subjects affected with Huntington's chorea who had been psychiatrically interviewed (B, Fig. 2)*

	Males (%) N = 40	Females (%) N = 61
Violence	21 (52·5)	13 (21·5)
Marital disorder*	11 (27·5)	4 (6·6)
Criminal offence	5 (12·5)	0
Alcoholism	3 (7·5)	0

* Separation or divorce.

Three male subjects tried to kill a spouse or child. There were nine cases of sexual disorder comprising incest two, rape two, exposure and transvestism three, all committed by male patients. Of these, four subjects were convicted and three more detained in a special hospital. There was no report of homosexual involvement.

3.1.7 Onset of functional psychiatric disorder in relation to the onset of Huntington's chorea

Fig. 13 shows the duration in years between the onset of functional psychiatric illness and personality disorder and the onset of physical signs of Huntington's chorea for the 65 subjects (Tables 9 and 10) in the psychiatrically interviewed section (C, Fig. 2) of the representative sample. The period of onset of Huntington's chorea is prolonged due to its insidious course with premonitory symptoms which are indeterminate for diagnosis. It was therefore decided that an illness or personality disorder commencing within 2 years before or two years after the onset of physical signs of Huntington's chorea would be assessed as within the period of onset. It can be seen (Fig. 13) that the onsets of

minor depression, behaviour and personality disorder cluster around the onset of Huntington's chorea while those of major depression and schizophrenia are more evenly distributed over a more extended time period. A comparison of variance (F ratio, Fisher, 1946) between diagnostic groups in respect of the period between their onsets and the physical onset of Huntington's chorea was calculated and the results in Fig. 13 show the onset of minor depression and personality disorder occurs significantly more frequently within the 4 years around the period of onset of Huntington's chorea than major depression and schizophrenia for which onset is distributed more widely and evenly over the period surveyed, i.e. before, during and after the onset of physical signs of Huntington's chorea. It can be assumed from this that minor depression and behaviour disorder are significantly associated with the onset of physical signs of Huntington's chorea while major depression and schizophrenia are not.

3.2 Subjects at an initial 50% risk for Huntington's chorea

Subjects at initial 50% risk were unaffected, living offspring and siblings of affected persons from the 34 kindreds of Section C (Fig. 2).

3.2.1 Age

There were 144 subjects at risk with almost equal numbers of each sex. The mean age and range in 1988 is similar between the sexes (Table 13).

Table 13. *Mean age in 1988 of subjects at 50% initial risk for Huntington's chorea*

	Males	Females	Total
N	69	75	144
Mean age	33·5	33·1	33·3
Range	15–69	17–73	15–73

For 15 subjects age was not known. One subject died by suicide and the age at death (18) is included. All persons included here were from affected families from whom a member had been referred for genetic counselling and possible linkage testing for Huntington's chorea.

3.2.2 Affective disorder

Thirty-five per cent of subjects at an initial 50% risk give a history of depression, one-third of

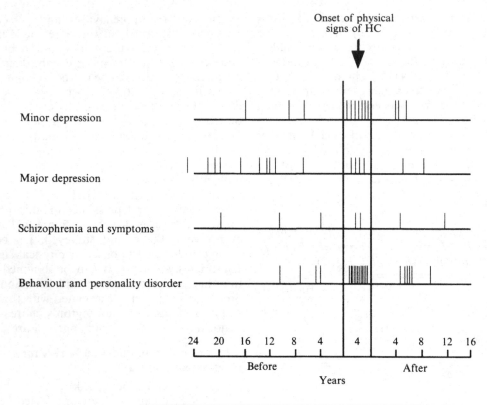

FIG. 13. The onset of functional psychiatric disorder before, after and simultaneously with the onset of Huntington's chorea. Variance of diagnostic categories compared.

Diagnosis compared		F ratio	
Schizophrenia	v. Personality disorder	4·54	P < 0·01
Schizophrenia	v. Minor depression	3·51	P < 0·05
Major depression	v. Personality disorder	4·19	P < 0·01
Major depression	v. Minor depression	3·24	P < 0·05

All tests are one-tailed.

which is major and two-thirds minor depression (Table 14). The figure for major depression is close to that for the general population (Table 18). Minor depressive illness affected about a quarter of both patients at initial 50% risk and those affected. A large number of these occurred coincidentally with severe stress: unemployment, divorce, death in the family, the onset of illness and the exigencies of care of an affected relative. The clinical impression that these illnesses are reactive is supported by the significant clustering

Table 14. *History of depression up to 1988 in subjects at 50% initial risk of Huntington's chorea*

	Males (%)	Females (%)	Total (%)
Minor depression	20·3	26·7	23·6
Major depression	13·3	9·3	11·1
Minor plus major depression	33·0	36·0	34·7
N	69	75	144

of their onsets around the onset of Huntington's chorea and their limited duration.

3.2.3 Other psychiatric disorders in 50% initial risk subjects

The only other diagnosis of adult psychiatric illness was schizo-affective disorder in a subject at risk aged 55. Three subjects were described as abnormally bad-tempered, but these were long-standing traits and not a change in temperament occurring in a mature, stable personality. No other initial 50% risk subjects gave a history of personality or behaviour disorder. It is notable that affected subjects had twice the frequency and a greater variety of types of functional psychiatric disorder than subjects at initial 50% risk, where it was confined to depressive disorder except for one case.

3.2.4 Comparison with conduct disorder in offspring of Huntington's chorea-affected patients

Our results can be compared with those of Folstein *et al.* (1983*a, b*) of the Maryland Huntington's disease project. Here functional psychiatric disorder was ascertained in 112 offspring of 34 subjects with Huntington's chorea. Twenty (18%)[1] were reported to have had major affective disorder and 28 (25%) had conduct disorder or antisocial personality. These are results from a population of relatives of subjects affected with Huntington's chorea who are themselves at initial 50% risk for developing it. In comparison with our population at initial 50% risk there is a considerable difference between their 26% of conduct disorder and our finding of no personality and behaviour disorder. This can be attributed mainly to the differences in the populations studied. The Maryland population consisted entirely of offspring of living affected subjects whereas our population contained a high proportion of siblings, which would considerably increase their mean age. More than 50% of these siblings lived in a family without a cohabiting affected person and the consequent family disturbance. That conduct and behaviour disorder was significantly related to disorganization of the affected parent's families is a notable result of Folstein *et al.*'s investigation (1983*a*). In addition all those

affected with conduct disorder were adolescents, in seven of whom the disorder recovered.

In contrast to Folstein *et al.*'s nosology (1983*a*), our categorization of personality and behaviour disorder required that a change took place in a mature and settled personality, which excluded behaviour disorders of childhood and adolescence. Had this not been so, three initial 50% risk subjects who were abnormally bad-tempered could have been categorized as personality disorder.

3.2.5 Comparison with controls (spouses)

In order to ascertain the effect of the presence of the Huntington gene on the development of functional psychiatric disorder, subjects at an initial 50% risk were compared with their spouses who shared their family environment, but did not have the Huntington's gene. Controls were available for slightly less than half the number of at risk subjects for reasons shown in Table 15. There is no material difference in the mean or range of age of subjects at initial 50% risk and controls (Table 16), so that the period of exposure to risk of functional psychiatric disorder did not differ between the two groups.

Table 15. *Subjects at 50% initial risk for developing Huntington's chorea for whom no controls (spouses) were available*

Single	43
Widowed	3
Separated/widowed	8
Not interviewed	11
Other	9
Total	74

Table 16. *Mean age and range of subjects at 50% initial risk of developing Huntington's chorea and their cohabiting spouses × sex*

	Subjects at 50% risk			Controls	
	Mean	Range	N = 66	Mean	Range
Females N = 36	40·1	21–58	Females N = 30	38·1	23–64
Males N = 30	36·8	22–69	Males N = 36	37·1	21–58

Controls were the spouses of subjects at risk. The unmarried, widowed, separated and divorced were not included.

[1] There is a slight discrepancy between these figures in the two reports of this study; 1983*a* is quoted here.

The distribution of functional psychiatric illness among subjects and controls is shown in Table 17. Functional psychiatric illness is significantly more frequent in subjects at 50% initial risk than in the zero risk controls ($\chi^2 = 8.447$, $P < 0.01$).

Table 17. *Functional psychiatric illness among subjects at 50% initial risk for Huntington's chorea and cohabiting spouses*

	50% risk ($N = 144$)	Controls ($N = 70$)
Total psychiatric illness	35%	13%
Minor depression	24%	10%
Major depression	11%	1%

These figures are consistent with an effect of the Huntington gene in that approximately 35% of the at risk group produced depression, whereas the results for spouses are at about the same level as for the general population (Table 20). However, other possible factors must be taken into account. First, the result for controls must be treated with caution as about a third of them could not be interviewed and we were reliant on report from the spouse. Secondly, the at risk group knew their status and most had intimate experience of the nature of the illness from at least a parent with Huntington's chorea and their reaction to this could contribute to their more frequent illness.

3.2.6 Predictive test results

Thirty-four families were referred for linkage testing but no results were obtained for 19 individuals for reasons shown in Table 18. The

Table 18. *Reasons for lack of test result in psychiatrically interviewed families*

Members of family at 50% risk did not wish to proceed with test	9
Pedigree not sufficiently informative	2
Family haplotypes uninformative	3
Blood (DNA) not available*	1
Test uninformative	2
50% risk subjects aged over 60†	2
Total	19

* Family member died before blood was obtained.
† Other members of the family of one of these subjects received a test result.

Table 19. *The frequency of functional psychiatric illness in subjects with a high probability of developing Huntington's chorea compared with those with low probability*

	Subjects having any functional psychiatric illness	Subjects having no functional psychiatric illness
High probability (gene carrier)	7 (37%)	12 (63%)
Low probability (non-gene carrier)	16 (47%)	18 (53%)
	$N = 53$	

test results indicated that 19 subjects had a high probability ($> 95\%$) and 34 subjects a low probability ($< 5\%$) of contracting Huntington's chorea. Table 19 shows the subjects for whom a linkage test result was obtained, sorted according to whether or not they had a history of functional psychiatric disorder (mainly depressive illness). No subject at initial 50% risk showed personality and behaviour disorder. It shows that similar proportions of the two probability groups had a positive functional psychiatric history ($\chi^2 = 0.4992$, $P > 0.1$), indicating that carriers of the Huntington gene did not show a greater tendency to functional psychiatric disorder than non-carriers of the gene who share a similar environment.

3.2.7 Comparison of prevalence of functional psychiatric disorder in subjects affected with Huntington's chorea with that in subjects at 50% initial risk for Huntington's chorea and also in other conditions

Table 20 shows the frequency of functional psychiatric disorder for subjects at 50% initial risk for Huntington's chorea compared with subjects affected with Huntington's chorea. The frequency of minor depression is about equal in the two groups, and of major depression the frequency in the affected group is about twice that in the group at 50% risk (Table 20). The difference in mean age between these two groups, however, shows the affected subjects to have been at risk for functional psychiatric disorder for just over twice the period of subjects at an initial 50% risk. Calculation to compensate for this difference, however, is restrained by the evidence that over 80% of major depressive illness in affected subjects occurs before or at the

Table 20. *Comparison of the prevalence of functional psychiatric disorder in Huntington's chorea with that in subjects at 50% initial risk, Alzheimer's disease and the general population*

Source... Type of population...	Present study HC affected	Present study HC 50% risk	Folstein et al. (1981) HC affected, USA, Maryland	Mindham et al. (1985) HC affected	Mindham et al. (1985) Alzheimer's disease	Bebbington et al. (1981) Composite of 7 studies	New Haven M%	New Haven F%	Baltimore M%	Baltimore F%	St Louis M%	St Louis F%
N	65	144	136	27	27							
Mean age	51 years	33 years										
Minor depression	28%	24%	3%	—	—		3	4	1	3	2	5
Major depression	26%	11%	41%	—	—		4	9	2	5	3	8
Total depression	54%	35%	44%	44%	26%	Male 4–8% Female 8–15%						
Schizophrenia	12%	—	5%				1	3	1	2	1	1
Behaviour and personality disorder	42%	—	39%	Burns et al. (1990)* 59%	Burns et al. (1990)* 32%		4	1	5	1	5	1

General population: Robins et al. (1984) (Table 3) — New Haven, Baltimore, St Louis

* The figures from **Burns** et al. (1990) refer to patients assessed for aggression.

period of onset of Huntington's chorea (mean 44 years), as shown in Fig. 13. Folstein *et al.* (1987) similarly found from retrospective study that the mean age of onset of episodic depression in affected subjects was over 4 years earlier than the onset of motor symptoms. This predominance of early onset of depressive illness in affected persons will minimize the effect of the difference in period of risk between the two groups and we must conclude that major depression occurs more frequently in affected subjects than in subjects at an initial 50 % risk. Comparison with the affected group shows that behaviour and personality disorder is not found among 50 % risk subjects but affects approaching a half of the affected. The number of schizophrenics identified is too small to allow a comparison between the affected and at risk groups.

Table 20 shows also that lifetime prevalence of functional psychiatric illnesses of both affected and 50 % initial risk subjects exceed reported estimates of lifetime prevalence of these disorders in the general population (Robins *et al.* 1984). The Maryland survey of Folstein *et al.* (1987) and the study of Mindham *et al.* (1985) (affective disorder only) give lifetime prevalence in affected

subjects reasonably close to those of this study for total depression. However, Folstein *et al.* (1987) found the proportion of major depression to be much higher than minor in affected subjects, whereas in the present study they are roughly equal (C Fig. 2, Table 9). Schizophrenia and behaviour and personality disorder frequency estimates are close to each other in Folstein *et al.* (1987) and the present study. Mindham *et al.* (1985) showed an almost significant ($P = 0.06$) lower frequency of functional psychiatric disorder in Alzheimer's disease than in Huntington's chorea (Table 20). In view of the greater age and consequent longer exposure to the risk of psychiatric disorder in Alzheimer's disease they conclude that this demonstrates that affective morbidity is greater among subjects with Huntington's chorea than among those with Alzheimer's disease. Our estimate of prevalence of functional psychiatric disorder in Huntington's chorea subjects similarly exceeds Mindham *et al.*'s prevalence in Alzheimer's disease. Burns *et al.* (1990) found Huntington's choreics significantly more aggressive than subjects with Alzheimer's disease, and their aggressive outbursts were more severe.

Chapter 4

Discussion

4.1 REVERSE GENETICS

The technique of cloning any gene from its chromosomal location when the protein product is not known, commonly referred to as 'reverse genetics' or 'positional cloning', has already proven a successful strategy in many instances. For example, the gene for Duchenne muscular dystrophy located on the short arm of X chromosome and that for cystic fibrosis on chromosome 7 were isolated by this technique (Koenig *et al.* 1987; Kerem *et al.* 1989). The general approach in reverse genetics is first to obtain a subchromosomal location for the gene often by demonstrating linkage to a polymorphic marker whose map location is already known or could be discovered by other methods. Often cytogenetic abnormalities such as translocations which are uniquely associated with the disease can also help to define the subchromosomal localization. For example, two patients with neurofibromatosis type 1 (NF1) were observed to have a reciprocal chromosomal translocation involving the same part of chromosome 17. It was subsequently shown that in both cases the translocation occurred within the NF1 gene, thereby disrupting its expression. Once a subchromosomal localization for the gene has been defined, efforts are then made to isolate further polymorphic markers which by linkage studies can be shown to map closer to the disease locus. It is desirable to obtain close markers which can be shown to 'flank' the disease gene, that is lie on either side, thus defining the smallest gap in which the gene must lie. Once this has been achieved, various techniques of molecular biology are employed to isolate the gene in the region. These techniques, which include chromosome walking and jumping, sequencing to map the defined region completely, followed by a detailed search for the various hallmarks of genes, are described in many molecular textbooks (e.g. Strachan, 1992). Once a gene has been found it must be examined for the presence of a mutation(s) consistent with expression of the disease phenotype.

4.2 CURRENT KNOWLEDGE OF THE HUNTINGTON'S CHOREA LOCUS

It is 10 years since Gusella *et al.* (1983) demonstrated linkage of the DNA marker G8 to Huntington's chorea using an unusually large Venezuelan HC pedigree. The G8 marker, and hence HC gene, was subsequently mapped using a panel of somatic cell hybrids and *in situ* hybridization to near the tip (or telomere) of the short arm (p) of chromosome 4 in the sub-band 4p16.3 (Fig. 14). To date no chromosomal

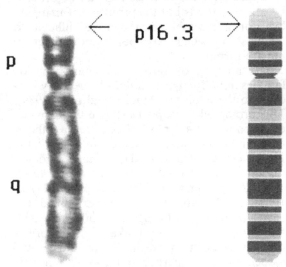

FIG. 14. Chromosome 4 and idiogram showing the cytogenetic sub-band p 16.3 in which the locus for Huntington's chorea resides. 'p' and 'q' are used to designate the short and long arms of the chromosome respectively.

rearrangement associated with the disease has been found, and linkage analysis has been the method employed to try to clone the gene.[1] Why is it taking so long? One reason is that DNA close to the telomere has been very difficult to work with, and although many markers have been isolated and have been shown to be more tightly linked to the HC gene than G8 none has been conclusively shown to map to the distal side of the gene.

[1] But see p. 39, for new information added during the preparation of this monograph.

When mapping loci the main problem is to obtain the correct order, which, even if every case is correctly diagnosed, is difficult. To order loci separated evenly at intervals such that there is a 1% chance of recombination (defined as 1 cM) between them requires more families than are available. The chance of an informative meiosis between any two loci, and on an average there is less than one per patient, is less than 1% per patient at the Huntington's chorea locus. In order to have a 50% chance of detecting a recombinant between any neighbouring loci 1 cM apart would require 70 cases (i.e. 0·99 to the power of 70 = 1/2 approximately) and this number of cases would have less than a 1/500 (i.e. 1/2 to the power of 9) chance of providing the necessary information to order 9 loci. Fortunately, some of these loci can be ordered by other methods but the problems of mapping loci for a disease which can be difficult to diagnose and which may not present until late in life are formidable.

The analysis of rare recombinants in HC families initially suggested that the gene lay very close to the telomere (MacDonald *et al.* 1989). This prompted attempts to isolate the telomere of chromosome 4p into a YAC, itself a difficult task. However, once achieved, analysis of the 115 kB clone failed to yield convincing evidence for the presence of the HC gene (Bates *et al.* 1990). At the same time other groups (Snell *et al.* 1989; Theilmann *et al.* 1989) examined the closer markers for linkage disequilibrium with the Huntington's gene. Linkage disequilibrium or allelic association is defined as the preferential association of a particular allele at a nearby locus (usually with a recombination fraction of less than 1%) more frequently than expected by chance. However, allelic association assumes a single mutation and even then the degree of association is poorly correlated with closeness of linkage. With two mutations in individuals leading to two types of families, different patterns of allelic association would be expected, notwithstanding the mutations being in the same place.

Allelic association was observed between Huntington's chorea and the markers D4S95 and D4S98 situated in the central region of the map (Fig. 15) but not with markers at either end of the map, with the markers D4S95 and D4S98 (see Fig. 15) situated in the central region of the

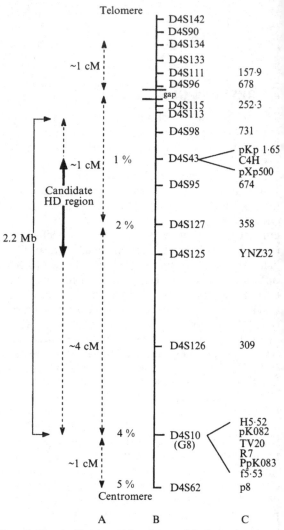

FIG. 15. Map showing the position of some of the loci and markers relative to the 2·2 Mb region thought to contain the Huntington's chorea gene as defined by Bates *et al.* (1991). A, Observed recombination fraction with HC; B, genetic loci; C, some of the polymorphic markers from within the identified loci – see Table 7 for details of markers used in this study.

map between G8 and the telomere, but was not observed with markers at either end of the map. Although the linkage disequilibrium data was not strong, it did not support a telomeric location for the HC gene and was in conflict with the linkage analysis of the rare recombinants, thus prompting reinvestigation of the recombinant pedigrees. Already further studies on these families (Bates *et al.* 1991; Pritchard *et al.* 1992) have produced new data which do not support a telomeric location for the HC gene and one of the suggestions is that at least in one of the families the HC gene may be located outside the region normally associated with HC in other families.

In summary, therefore, the present picture is confusing. Efforts are now being directed at searching a 2000 kb region around D4S95 locus for the gene. This region, however, could contain 40 or more genes and the work involved in characterizing these and demonstrating whether an observed mutation(s) could be responsible for the HC phenotype is immense. A further problem is that most proteins have more than one subunit, and the subunits usually have loci on different chromosomes, so that mistakes on different chromosomes may lead to very similar consequences. This has been shown to be the case for the two different forms of thalassaemia. The only two successes in gene isolation through linkage, cystic fibrosis and myotonic dystrophy, are caused by mutations involving a protein compounded of a single unit. This may take a further 10 years, unless there is astute clinical observation of related disorders or other types of variants, or (with luck) the gene could be found tomorrow.

[During the preparation of this monograph 'tomorrow' has arrived!]

In March 1993 the Huntington's Disease Collaborative Research Group published a paper in which they reported the isolation of a novel gene containing a trinucleotide repeat that is expanded and unstable on Huntington's disease chromosomes (The Huntington's Disease Collaborative Research Group, 1993). The 210-kilobase gene, known as IT15, encodes a 348K protein which appears to be unrelated to any existing protein in the databases. A polymorphic CAG trinucleotide repeat (i.e. the DNA sequence CAG repeated 'n' times) lies at the 5′ end of the gene which shows amplification in affected patients. There are at least 17 discrete alleles in the normal population ranging from 11–34 copies of the repeat whereas in patients with Huntington's disease alleles which range in size from 42 to over 66 copies have been observed. There is also apparent correlation with the age of onset, the largest expansions

being associated with juvenile onset of the disease. Trinucleotide repeat expansion has also recently been shown to be associated with the expression of three other genetic diseases; myotonic dystrophy, (Brook *et al.* 1992) fragile X (Kremer *et al.* 1991) and spino-bulbar muscular atrophy (La Spada *et al.* 1991), and may prove to be a common mechanism in human genetic disease.

It is at present unclear what the function of the normal 'Huntingtin' protein might be or how increase in trinucleotide repeat length results in the expression of Huntington's disease. There is evidence that the expanded trinucleotide repeat does not simply cause inactivation of the gene and it has been suggested that the altered protein may have new properties or that the presence of the expansion might directly affect the regulation, localization, or stability of translation of the mRNA containing it. The possibility also remains that although the repeat is located within the IT15 transcript, it may lead to Huntington's chorea by acting on the expression of another gene.

This exciting discovery has implications for the predictive test. In theory it should now be possible to provide accurate presymptomatic or prenatal diagnosis by assaying directly the size of the trinucleotide repeat in 'at risk' individuals, thereby eliminating the need for time-consuming linkage analysis. It should also be possible to extend predictive testing to individuals with no living affected relatives. However, while the current data implies that there is no overlap in the range of repeat length in normal alleles and Huntington's alleles and that there is a direct correlation between age of onset and size of the repeat, further studies are needed to confirm these findings. The Huntington's Disease Collaborative Research Group strongly urge that the existing internationally agreed protocols for presymptomatic and prenatal testing are followed until these studies are completed.

Thus, with the molecular basis of Huntington's chorea apparently resolved the next challenge is to understand the function of the Huntingtin protein and the pathogenesis of the disease, which it is hoped will lead one day to the successful treatment of this devastating condition.

4.3 PREVALENCE

The prevalence we have found of 40 persons affected with Huntington's chorea per million of the general population comes at the low end of the wide spectrum of reported results tabulated by Hayden (1981), Conneally (1984), Folstein (1989) and Harper (1991) and is close to that of Reed & Chandler (1958). The variation in these estimates is partly attributable to the clustering tendency of Huntington's chorea deriving from its familial mode of transmission, which is particularly prominent in geographical isolates as in Venezuela (Avila-Giron, 1973), Tasmania (Brothers, 1949) and in Harper's (1991) description of accumulation in a static population in Wales, all of which show a high prevalence. Only estimates of prevalence based on a large general population, at least a million, which is not geographically isolated, should be compared. The Oxford Health Region has a population of 2·5 million. All parts are easily accessible. It has regular genetic clinics in every town with a general hospital (Fig. 1) and its administration is in Oxford, which is central in the region.

Our estimates of the prevalence of psychiatric disorder in affected subjects are calculated from section C (Fig. 2) which is the 67% forming those whom we psychiatrically interviewed with their families from the total representative sample (A, Fig. 2) of those subjects affected with HC living in the Oxford Health Region in 1988. There is no significant difference in the distribution of means of the ages (Table 7) or in the distribution of sexes between these two groups. Thus, valid results from these populations may be generalized to other comparable populations.

4.4 GENETIC, ORGANIC AND ENVIRONMENTAL FACTORS BEARING ON PSYCHOPATHOLOGY OF FUNCTIONAL PSYCHIATRIC DISORDER

Three sections of our population can be distinguished according to the proportion in each carrying the Huntington's chorea gene. There are first, those who have no parent affected with Huntington's chorea, none of whom therefore carry an HC gene and who are therefore uniformly homozygotic. Secondly, individuals who are symptom-free but have a parent affected with Huntington's chorea have at birth a 50%

chance of carrying the HC gene and thus less than a 50% chance of developing Huntington's chorea, which declines with age. Populations of such individuals will average up to 50% of heterozygotes who are not clinically identifiable as such. If however the genetic linkage test is administered, a known proportion will probably be individually identified as asymptomatic heterozygotes. The third section consists of individuals all affected with Huntington's chorea 100% of whom are therefore heterozygotes. If the presence of the Huntington's chorea (HC) gene causes functional psychiatric disorder (fpd) the incidence of fpd in each of the three sections which we have distinguished would be similar to the proportion of HC genes in each section. That is, subjects of the first section (no HC gene, homozygotes) would show least fpd, the third section (all having an HC gene, heterozygotes) would show most and in the second (a proportion of subjects who were heterozygotes without physical symptoms of HC) the number with functional psychiatric disorder would be intermediate. These proportions of functional psychiatric disorder are in fact observed (Table 20). When, however, a correction is made for the difference between these groups in respect of the mean period of exposure to the risk of incurring functional psychiatric disorder, the proportions affected do not correspond to the proportions of heterozygotes, e.g. no individual functional psychiatric disorder affects 100% of the heterozygotes with or without Huntington's chorea, nor does functional psychiatric disorder as a whole have this effect: a proportion of HC gene carriers have no functional psychiatric disorder (Table 19). Therefore, the Huntington's chorea gene must be regarded at most as not fully penetrant for any functional psychiatric disorder.

4.5 MAJOR AND MINOR DEPRESSIVE ILLNESS

Although there is a considerable difference between our estimates of frequency of major and minor depressive illness and those of Folstein *et al.* (1983c) (Table 20), it is clear that major affective disorder constitutes the largest portion of functional psychiatric illness arising in Huntington's chorea. Folstein *et al.* (1983c) make the suggestion that major affective disorder 'could have been introduced by additional later mutations within the postulated Huntington's disease locus which produces the more complex Huntington disease/affective disorder phenotype'. There would thus be two alleles of Huntington's chorea gene, one of which additionally produced major affective illness, and Huntington's chorea would in this respect be genetically heterogeneous. This hypothesis seems unlikely, however, in that it presents a mechanism hitherto unknown in genetics. A further mutation in a locus already producing a disease usually results in a more severe form of the same disease, as in the fragile X syndrome and myotonic dystrophy, if any change occurs. Furthermore, it is not supported by our comparison showing no significant difference in the proportion of subjects with functional psychiatric disorder in homozygotes against that in heterozygotes, both identified among asymptomatic offspring of Huntington's choreic parents by the genetic linkage test (Table 19). In Table 19 the homozgyotes (without HC gene) have slightly more functional psychiatric disorder than the heterozygotes (with HC gene) indicating clearly that the effect of the presence of the Huntington's gene is not to produce more functional psychiatric disorder (mainly depressive) than its absence in asymptomatic subjects at 50 % initial risk. Two objections to this conclusion might be raised. First, that the gene might not produce functional psychiatric disorder until it has shown its activity by producing Huntington's chorea. In fact, however, we found that the onset of the most major depressive illnesses preceded the onset of chorea (Fig. 3). Secondly, it might be suggested that the number of tested subjects (53) is too small to give a reliable, generalizable result. This seems unlikely, but a firm answer must await larger numbers and confirmation from other data.

Other evidence of morbid change to which depression might be attributed has been demonstrated in the pre-symptomatic stage of Huntington's chorea by brain scanning and neuropsychological tests. The former indicates that for up to 5 years before the onset of physical signs and psychological symptoms evidence of brain pathology in the form of reduced glucose metabolism is found in the basal ganglia by PET scan (Hayden *et al.* 1986; Hosokawa *et al.* 1987;

Mazziota *et al.* 1987). Jason *et al.* (1988) compared seven 50 % initial risk subjects having positive results from pre-symptomatic linkage testing (i.e. carrying the Huntington's chorea gene) with three 50 % initial risk subjects having negative results and showed a significant deficit in visuospatial memory and in specific functions associated with frontal lobes in predicted carriers, whereas predicted non-carriers were free of such impairment. Neither group demonstrated impairment of general intelligence, language ability, verbal memory, manual dexterity or tapping speed, thus showing conclusively no onset of clinical signs of Huntington's chorea. There is no evidence that subjects are aware of these processes in any way which would reveal their significance and therefore no reason for them to produce a reactive depression. The structural and functional brain damage revealed by these two methods might operate as an organic cause of major depression but, in fact, no clustering of onset of major depression in the first 5 years before onset of Huntington's chorea is shown in Fig. 13.

That cerebral damage and the social disorder in families attributable to Huntington's chorea produce other functional psychiatric disorder, however, seems undoubted and is not unexpected. The tendency of the onset of personality and behaviour disorder and of minor depressive illness to cluster about the onset of Huntington's chorea (Fig. 3) suggest that these disorders are more subject to and significantly produced by these influences. The cases of heterozygotes living in HC families quoted by Dewhurst (1970) who produced personality and behaviour disorder, and the demonstration by Folstein *et al.* (1983 *a*) of its correlation with family disorder in the offspring of Huntington's choreics, also support this view.

Patients' awareness of the onset of Huntington's chorea is also likely to be a potent influence in producing depression. Mindham *et al.* (1981), for instance, demonstrated the presence of depression as a severe, active disease which seriously interfered with daily activities in patients with rheumatoid arthritis. Brown *et al.* (1988) found depression in the course of Parkinson's disease which showed close correlation in severity with the level of disability. Patients realizing the onset of Huntington's chorea have usually had a powerful demonstration of its effects in the illness of a parent and other relatives.

The amount of functional psychiatric disorder (predominantly depression) found in cohabiting spouses of subjects at 50% initial risk (Table 17) is close to that found in the general population (Table 20).

4.6 SCHIZOPHRENIA

The fact that so little schizophrenia occurred among subjects at 50% initial risk makes the number of tested subjects too small to show whether an increased risk of schizophrenia occurs in association with the Huntington's chorea gene, but suggests that its effect cannot at any rate be large. The number of schizophrenics included in our comparison of time of onset with that of Huntington's chorea is also small, and conclusions are therefore tentative. Nevertheless, the onset of schizophrenia appears evenly distributed independently of the stage of Huntington's chorea, suggesting no connection between the two. Davison (1983) reports Huntington's chorea among the heterogeneous group of diseases and conditions in which a schizophrenia-like syndrome occurs. This list is extended by the genetic and CNS diseases, pharmacological and toxic substances reviewed by Propping (1983) as producing schizophrenia. We must add as well the considerable number of schizophrenics found with organic brain diseases. Kay (1963), for instance, has convincingly shown age-dependent specific brain impairments to be related to the frequency of onset of schizophrenia. All these conditions share the characteristic of a partial and generalized unpredictable schizophrenogenic effect, which implies as a substrate a variable diathesis such as would arise as described by Pearson (1904), Edwards (1960, 1969, 1972), Falconer (1965) and Gottesman & Shields (1972).

4.7 BEHAVIOUR AND PERSONALITY DISORDER

Behaviour and personality disorder is the most frequent psychiatric condition we have found in association with Huntington's chorea. Their definition was described as the least satisfactory section of the WHO programme on Psychiatric Diagnosis (Shepherd & Sartorius, 1974). We have followed its recommendation that 'if this [disorder] is determined primarily by malfunctioning of the brain it should...be classified...as one of the non-psychotic brain syndromes' and for further categorization we have used the most prominent characteristic of the behaviour or attitude.

Aggressiveness is the most frequent functional psychiatric condition occurring in Huntington's chorea, manifesting in over half the males and almost half of the females. Suspiciousness and temper occur in between a quarter and a third of both (Table 11). In a comparison with Alzheimer's disease, Burns *et al.* (1990) demonstrate that Huntington's chorea produces a significantly more severe and prolonged type of aggression and this probably makes it outstanding among brain disorders in this respect.

Fig. 3 shows a prominent tendency of personality and behaviour disorders to have their onset during or in the first period after the onset of Huntington's chorea which, of the disorders which we are considering, ties them most directly to brain pathology. However, the examples we have quoted from Dewhurst (1970) of behaviour disorder occurring in spouses and other unrelated members of the family group with zero risk of contracting HC, of Huntington's choreics and Folstein *et al.*'s (1983*a, b*) study of effects on the behaviour of their offspring must remind us that the family disorder frequently seen in Huntington's chorea may produce a temporary disorder of conduct in individual family members living together.

4.8 CONCLUSIONS

Asymptomatic heterozygotes appear to have no functional psychiatric disorder produced by the Huntington's gene, a conclusion, however, that must remain tentative until confirmed by a larger number of results from linkage-tested subjects. It appears that personality and behaviour disorder are produced by brain damage and family disorder; and minor depression by reaction to the minatory and destructive effect of Huntington's chorea on the ordered life of the family, the individual and offspring.

Counselling 50% initial risk subjects on alternatives to producing their own children is likely to be made more effective by the application of linkage testing, which would result in concentrating counselling on those with a high probability of developing Huntington's chorea. In view of the surprisingly large number (12% in this study, Table 18) of eligible subjects who decline the offer of a linkage test, it might be profitable to emphasize the value of this strategy in reducing the incidence of Huntington's chorea when counselling subjects at risk and including it in general medical and lay information.

In view of prominent manifestation of major depressive disorder in both affected (28%) and in those at 50% initial risk (11%) it should be borne in mind that Folstein *et al.* (1979) and others have demonstrated clinically that major depressive illness appears as responsive to specific treatment as it is in the general population.

Our study has revealed points at which the study of functional psychiatric syndromes in Huntington's chorea might yield more information of which schizophrenia is the most striking example. Here, the lifetime prevalence yielded only 7 cases of schizophrenia from affected subjects and one schizo-affective from subjects at 50% initial risk, which allows neither a fruitful comparison of these two populations nor of the populations with positive and negative test results to ascertain the role of the Huntington's chorea gene. Of 199 cases of Huntington's chorea in the study of Saugstad & Ødegård, (1986) from Norway, 20% were discharged from first admission to a psychiatric hospital with a diagnosis of schizophrenia. This ascertainment was made using a psychiatric National Case Register which seems the most suitable method of collecting a large enough number of cases to test the effect of the Huntington's chorea gene in the production of schizophrenia.

REFERENCES

American Psychiatric Association (1980). *Diagnostic and Statistical Manual of Mental Disorders (DSM-III)*. APA: Washington, DC.

American Psychiatric Association (1987). *Diagnostic and Statistical Manual of Mental Disorders (3rd edn, revised) (DSM-III-R)*. APA: Washington, DC.

Avila-Giron, R. (1973). Medical and social aspects of Huntington's chorea in the state of Zulia, Venezuela. In *Huntington's Chorea 1872–1972* (ed. A. Barbeau, T. N. Chase and G. W. Paulson), pp. 261–266. Raven Press: New York.

Bakker, E., Skraastad, M. I., Fisser-Groen, Y. M., van Ommen, G. J. B. & Pearson, P. L. (1987). Two additional RFLPs at the D4S10 locus, useful for Huntington's disease (HD) – family studies. *Nucleic Acid Research* 15, 9100.

Bates, G. P., MacDonald, M. E., Baxendale, S., Sedlackek, Z., Youngman, S., Romano, D., Whaley, W. L., Allito, B., Poustka, A., Gusella, J. & Lehrach, H. (1990). A yeast artificial chromosome telomere clone spanning a positive location of the Huntington disease gene. *American Journal of Human Genetics* 46, 762–779.

Bates, G. P., MacDonald, M. E., Baxendale, S., Youngman, S., Lin, C., Whalley, W. L., Wasmuth, J. J., Gusella, J. F. & Lehrach, H. (1991). Defined physical limits of the Huntington's disease gene candidate region. *American Journal of Human Genetics* 49, 7–16.

Bebbington, P., Hurry, J., Tennant, C., Sturt, E. & Wing, J. (1981). Epidemiology of mental disorders in Camberwell. *Psychological Medicine* 11, 561–579.

Bell, J. (1948). Huntington's chorea. *Treasury of Human Inheritance*, Vol. 4 (ed. R. A. Fisher and L. S. Penrose), pp. 1–29. Cambridge University Press: Cambridge.

Bickford, J. A. R. & Ellison, R. M. (1953). The high incidence of Huntington's chorea in the Duchy of Cornwall. *Journal of Mental Science* 99, 291–294.

Boll, T. J., Heaton, R. & Reiton, R. M. (1971). Neuropsychological and emotional correlates of Huntington's chorea. *Journal of Nervous and Mental Diseases* 153, 61–69.

Bolt, J. M. W. (1970). Huntington's chorea in the west of Scotland. *British Journal of Psychiatry* 116, 259–270.

Brook, J. D., McCurrach, M. E., Harley, H. G., Buckler, A. J., Church, D. C., Aburatani, H., Hunter, K., Stanton, V. P., Thirion, J. P., Hudson, T., Sohn, R., Zemelman, B., Snell, R. G., Rundle, S. A., Crow, S., Davies, J., Shelbourne, S. A., Buxton, J., Jones, C., Juvonen, V., Johnson, K., Harper, P. S., Shaw, D. J. & Housman, D. E. (1992). Molecular basis of myotonic dystrophy: expansion of a trinucleotide repeat at the 3'- end of a transcript encoding a protein kinase family member. *Cell* 68, 799–808.

Brothers, C. R. D. (1949). The history and incidence of Huntington's chorea in Tasmania. *Proceedings of the Royal Australian College of Physicians* 4, 48–50.

Brothers, C. R. D. (1964). Huntington's chorea in Victoria and Tasmania. *Journal of Neurological Science* 1, 405–420.

Brothers, C. R. D. & Meadows, A. W. (1955). An investigation of Huntington's chorea in Victoria. *Journal of Mental Science* 101, 548–563.

Brown, R. G., MacCarthy, B., Gotham, A-M., Der, G. J. & Marsden, C. D. (1988). Depression and disability in Parkinson's disease – a follow-up of 132 cases. *Psychological Medicine* 18, 49–55.

Burns, A., Folstein, S., Braneth, J. & Folstein, M. (1990). Clinical assessment of irritability, aggression and apathy in Huntington and Alzheimer Disease. *Journal of Nervous and Mental Disease* 178, 20–26.

Caine, E. D. & Shoulson, I. (1983). Psychiatric syndromes in Huntington's disease. *American Journal of Psychiatry* 140, 728–733.

Caro, A. (1977). A genetic problem in East Anglia: Huntington's chorea. M.D. thesis, University of East Anglia.

Caro, A. (1993). Personal communication.

Chandler, J. H., Reed, T. E. & DeJong, R. N. (1960). Huntington's chorea in Michigan. III. Clinical observations. *Neurology* 10, 148–153.

Conneally, P. M. (1984). Huntington disease: genetics and epidemiology. *American Journal of Human Genetics* 36, 506–526.

Crauford, D. & Tyler, A. (1992). Predictive testing for Huntington's disease: protocol of the UK Huntington's prediction consortium. *Journal of Medical Genetics* 29, 915–918.

Dalby, S. (1986). A presymptomatic test for Huntington's chorea. Association to Combat Huntington's Chorea (COMBAT; now Huntington's Disease Association, 108 Battersea High Street, London SW11 3HP).

Davenport, C. B. & Muncey, E. B. (1916). Huntington's chorea in relation to heredity and eugenics. *American Journal of Insanity* 73, 195–222.

Davies, K. E. & Read, A. P. (1988). *Molecular Basis of Inherited Disease*. IRL Press: Oxford.

Davison, K. (1983). Schizophrenia-like psychoses associated with organic cerebral disorders: a review. *Psychiatric Developments* 1, 1–34.

Dewhurst, K. (1970). Personality disorder in Huntington's disease. *Psychiatrica Clinica* 3, 221–229.

Dewhurst, K., Oliver, J., Trick, K. L. K. & McKnight, A. L. (1969). Neuro-psychiatric aspects of Huntington's disease, *Confinia Neurologica* 31, 255–258.

Dewhurst, K., Oliver, J. E. & McKnight, A. L. (1970). Sociopsychiatric consequences of Huntington's disease. *British Journal of Psychiatry* 116, 258–268.

Dunlap, C. B. (1927). Pathologic changes in Huntington's chorea with special reference to the corpus striatum. *Archives of Neurology and Psychiatry* 18, 867–943.

Edwards, J. H. (1960). The simulation of Mendelism. *Acta Genetica* 10, 63–70.

Edwards, J. H. (1969). Familial predisposition in man. *British Medical Bulletin* 25, 58–64.

Edwards, J. H. (1972). The genetical basis of schizophrenia. In *Genetic Factors in 'Schizophrenia'* (ed. A. R. Kaplan), pp. 310–313. Thomas: Illinois.

Falconer, D. S. (1965). The inheritance of liability to certain diseases, estimated from the incidence among relatives. *Annals of Human Genetics* 29, 51–76.

Fisher, R. A. (1946). *Statistical Methods for Research Workers*, 10th edn. Oliver & Boyd: Edinburgh.

Folstein, M. F. & McHugh, P. R. (1983). The neuropsychiatry of some specific brain disorders. In *Handbook of Psychiatry*, vol. 2. *Mental Disorders and Somatic Illness* (ed. M. H. Lader), pp. 107–118. Cambridge University Press: Cambridge.

Folstein, S. E. (1989). *Huntington's Disease: A Disorder of Families*, p. 60. Johns Hopkins University Press: Baltimore.

Folstein, S. E. & Folstein, M. F. (1983). Psychiatric features of Huntington's disease: recent approaches and findings. *Psychiatric Developments* 2, 193–206

Folstein, S. E., Folstein, M. F. & McHugh, P. R. (1979). Psychiatric syndromes in Huntington's disease. In *Advances in Neurology* (ed. T. N. Chase, N. Wexler and A. Barbeau) 23, pp. 281–289. Raven Press: New York.

Folstein, S. E., Franz, M. L., Jensen, B. A., Chase, G. A. & Folstein, M. F. (1983a). Conduct disorder and affective disorder among offspring of patients with Huntington's disease. *Psychological Medicine* 13, 45–52.

Folstein, S. E., Franz, M. L., Jensen, B., Chase, G. A. & Folstein, M.F. (1983b). Conduct disorder and affective disorder among the offspring of patients with Huntington's disease. In *Childhood Psychopathology and Development* (ed. S. B. Guze, F. J. Earls and J. E. Barret), pp. 231–246. Raven Press: New York.

Folstein, S. E., Abbot, M. H., Chase, G. A., Jensen, B. A. & Folstein, M. F. (1983c). The association of affective disorder with Huntington's disease: in a case series and in families. *Psychological Medicine* 13, 537–542.

Folstein, S. E., Leigh, R. J., Parhard, I. M. & Folstein, M. F. (1986). The diagnosis of Huntington's disease. *Neurology* 36, 1279–83.

Folstein, S. E., Abbot, M., Moser, R., Parhad, I., Clark, A. & Folstein, M. F. (1987). Huntington's disease in Maryland: clinical aspects of racial variation. *American Journal of Human Genetics* 41, 168–179.

Fox, S., Bloch, M., Fahy, M. & Hayden, M. R. (1989). Predictive testing for Huntington disease. I. Description of a pilot project in British Columbia. *American Journal of Medical Genetics* 32, 211–216.

Goldberg, D. (1972). *The Detection of Psychiatric Illness by Questionnaire. Maudsley Monograph, No. 21.* Oxford University Press: Oxford.

Gottesman, I. I. & Shields, J. (1972). *Schizophrenia and Genetics.* Academic Press. New York.

Gusella, J. F., Wexler, N. S., Conneally, P. M., Naylor, S. L., Anderson, M. A., Tanzi, R. E., Watkins, P. C., Ottina, K., Wallace, M. R., Sakaguchi, A. Y., Young, A. B., Shoulson, I., Bonilla, E. & Martin, J. B. (1983). A polymorphic DNA marker genetically linked to Huntington's disease. *Nature* 306, 234–238.

Harper, P. S. (1991). The epidemiology of Huntington's disease. In *Huntington's Disease* (ed. P. Harper), pp. 251–280. W. B. Saunders: London.

Harper, P. S. Walker, D. A., Tyler, A., Newcombe, R. G. & Davies, K. (1979). Huntington's chorea. The basis for long-term prevention. *Lancet* ii, 346–349.

Hayden, M. R. (1981). *Huntington's Chorea.* Springer: Berlin.

Hayden, M. R., MacGregor, J. M. & Beighton, P. H. (1980). The prevalence of Huntington's chorea in South Africa. *South African Medical Journal* 58, 193–196.

Hayden, M. R., Martin, W. R. W., Stoessl, A. J., Clark, C., Hollenberg, S., Adam, M. J., Amman, W., Harrop, R., Rogers, J., Ruth, T., Sayre, C. & Pate, B. D. (1986). Positron emission tomography in the early diagnosis of Huntington's disease. *Neurology* 36, 888–894.

Hayden, M. R., Kastelein, J. P. P., Wilson, R. P., Hilbert, C., Hewitt, J., Langley, S., Fox, S. & Bloch, M. (1987a). First trimester prenatal diagnosis for Huntington's disease with DNA probes. *Lancet* i, 1284–1285.

Hayden, M. R., Hewitt, J., Martin, W. R. W., Clark, G. & Amman, W. (1987b). Studies in persons at risk for Huntington's disease. *New England Journal of Medicine* 317, 382–383.

Hayden, M. R., Hewitt, J., Stoessl, M. D., Clark, C., Amman, W. & Martin, W. R. W. (1987c). The combined use of positron emission tomography and DNA polymorphisms for preclinical detection of Huntington's disease. *Neurology* 37, 1441–1447.

Heathfield, K. W. G. (1968). Huntington's chorea: investigation into the prevalence of this disease in the area covered by the N.E. Metropolitan Regional Board. *Brain* 90, 203–232.

Hosokawa, S., Ichiya, Y., Kuwabara, Y., Ayabe, Z., Mitsuo, K., Goto, I., Kato, M. (1987). Positron emission tomography in cases of chorea with different underlying diseases. *Journal of Neurology and Psychiatry* 50, 1284–1287.

Hughes, E. M. (1925). Social significance of Huntington's chorea. *American Journal of Psychiatry* 4, 537–574.

Huntington's Disease Collaborative Research Group (1993). A novel gene containing a trinucleotide repeat that is expanded and unstable on Huntington's disease chromosomes. *Cell* 72, 971–983.

Jason, G. W., Pajurkova, E. M., Suchowersky, O., Hewitt, J., Hilbert, C., Reed, J. & Hayden, M. (1988). Presymptomatic neuropsychological impairment in Huntington's disease. *Archives of Neurology* 45, 769–773.

Kay, D. W. K. (1963). Late paraphrenia and its bearing on the aetiology of schizophrenia. *Acta Psychiatrica Scandinavica* 39, 159–169.

Kerem, B., Rommens, J., Buchanan, J., Markiewicz, D., Cox, T. K.,

Chakravarti, A., Buchwald, M. & Tsui, L-C. (1989). Identification of the cystic fibrosis gene: genetic analysis. *Science* 245, 1073–1080.

King, M. (1985). Alcohol abuse in Huntington's chorea. *Psychological Medicine* 15, 815–820.

Kishimoto, K., Nakamura, M. & Sotokawa, Y. (1957). Population genetics study of Huntington's chorea in Japan. *Annual Report of the Research Institute of Environmental Medicine* 9, 195–211.

Koenig, M., Hoffman, E. P., Bertelson, C. J., Monaco, A. P., Feener, C. & Kunkel, L. M. (1987). Complete cloning of the Duchenne muscular dystrophy gene. *Cell* 50, 509–517.

Kremer, E. J., Pritchard, M., Lynch, M., Yu, S., Holman, K., Baker, E., Warren, S. T., Schlessinger, D., Sutherland, G. R. & Richards, R. I. (1991). Mapping of DNA instability at the fragile X to a trinucleotide repeat sequence p(CCG)n. *Science* 252, 1711–1714.

La Spada, A. R., Wilson, E. M., Lubahn, D., Harding, A. E. & Fishbeck, K. H. (1991). Androgen receptor gene mutations in X-linked spinal and bulbar muscular atrophy. *Nature* 352, 77–79.

Lewis, A. (1971). 'Endogenous' and 'exogenous': a useful dichotomy? *Psychological Medicine* 1, 191–196.

Lilienfeld, A. M. & Lilienfeld, D. E. (1980). *Foundations of Epidemiology,* 2nd edn. Oxford University Press: Oxford.

MacDonald, M. E., Cheng, S. V., Zimmer, M., Haines, H. L., Poustka, A., Allitto, B. A., Smith, B., Whaley, W. L., Romano, D., Jagadesh, J., Myers, R., Lehrach, H., Wasmuth, J. J., Frischauf, A. & Gusella, J. (1989a). Clustering of multi-allele DNA markers near the Huntington's disease gene. *Journal of Clinical Investigation* 84, 1013–1016.

MacDonald, M. E., Haines, H. L., Zimmer, M., Cheng, S. V., Youngman, S., Whaley, W. L., Allito, B., Smith, B., Leavitt, J., Poustka, A., Harper, P., Lehrach, H., Wasmuth, J. J., Frischauf, A. & Gusella, J. (1989b). Recombination events suggest potential sites for the Huntington's disease gene. *Neuron* 3, 183–190.

McHugh, P. R. & Folstein, M. F. (1975). Psychiatric syndromes of Huntington's chorea: a clinical and phenomenological study. In *Psychiatric Aspects of Neurologic Disease* (ed. D. F. Benson and D. Blumer), pp. 267–286. Grune & Stratton: New York.

Markowe, M., Steinert, J. & Heyworth-Davies, F. (1967). Insulin and chlorpromazine in schizophrenia: a ten-year comparative survey. *British Journal of Psychiatry* 113, 1101–1106.

Marsden, C. D. (1982). Basal ganglia disease. *Lancet* ii, 1141–1147.

Martello, N., Santos, J. L. F. & Frota-Pessoa, O. (1978). Risks of manifestation of Huntington's chorea. *Journal de Génétique Humaine* 26, 33–53.

Mattsson, B. (1974a). Huntington's chorea in Sweden. I. Prevalence and genetic data. *Acta Psychiatrica Scandinavica* suppl. 255, 211–220.

Mattsson, B. (1974b). Huntington's chorea in Sweden. II. Social and clinical data. *Acta Psychiatrica Scandinavica* suppl. 255, 221–236.

Mayer-Gross, W., Slater, E. & Roth, M. (1954). *Clinical Psychiatry.* Cassell: London.

Mazziota, J. C., Phelps, M. E., Pahl, J. J., Sung-cheng, H., Lewis, B. B., Riege, W. H., Hoffman, J. M., Kuhl, D. E., Lanto, A. B., Wapenski, J. A. & Markham, C. H. (1987). Reduced cerebral glucose metabolism in asymptomatic subjects at risk for Huntington's disease. *New England Journal of Medicine* 316, 357–362.

Mindham, R. H. S., Bagshaw, A., James, S. A. & Swannell, A. J. (1981). Factors associated with the appearance of rheumatoid arthritis. *Journal of Psychosomatic Research* 25, 429–435.

Mindham, R. H. S., Steele, C., Folstein, M. F. & Lucas, J. (1985). A comparison of the frequency of major affective disorder in Huntington's disease and Alzheimer's disease. *Journal of Neurology, Neurosurgery and Psychiatry* 48, 1172–1174.

Myers, J. K., Weissman, M. M., Tischler, G. L., Holzer, C. E., Leaf, P. J., Orvaschel, H. A., Boyd, J. H., Burke, J. D., Kramer, M. & Stoltzman, R. (1984). Six month prevalence of psychiatric disorders in three communities. *Archives of General Psychiatry* 41, 959–967.

Myrianthopoulos, N. C. (1973). Huntington's chorea: the genetic problem five years later. In *Huntington's Chorea, 1872–1972* (ed. A. Barbeau, T. M. Chase and G. W. Paulson), pp. 150–152. Raven Press: New York.

Neophytides, A. N., Di Chiro, G., Barron, S. A. & Chase, T. N. (1979). Computed axial tomography in Huntington's disease and persons at risk for Huntington's disease. *Advances in Neurology* 23, 185–191.

Oliver, J. E. (1970). Huntington's chorea in Northamptonshire. *British Journal of Psychiatry* 116, 241–253.

Oliver, J. E. & Dewhurst, K. E. (1969). Six generations of ill-used children in a Huntington's pedigree. *Postgraduate Medical Journal* 45, 757–760.

Padberg, G. & Bruyn, G. W. (1986). Chorea: differential diagnosis. In *Handbook of Clinical Neurology*, vol. 49 (ed. P. R. Vinken, G. W. Bruyn & H. L. Klemans), pp. 549–564. Elsevier: Amsterdam

Panse, F. (1942). *Erbchorea: eine Klinisch-genetische Studie*. Thieme: Leipzig.

Parker, N. (1958). Observations on Huntington's chorea based on a Queensland survey. *Medical Journal of Australia* 1, 251–259.

Pearson, K. (1904). On the laws of inheritance in man. II. On the inheritance of mental and moral characters in man and its comparison with the inheritance of the physical characters. *Biometrika* 3, 131–190.

Pearson, J. S., Peterson, M. C., Lazarte, J. A., Blodgett, H. E. & Key, I. B. (1955). An educational approach to the social problem of Huntington's chorea. *Proceedings of Staff Meetings of the Mayo Clinic* 30, 349–357.

Pflanz, S., Besson, J. A. O., Ebmeier, K. P. & Simpson, S. (1991). The clinical manifestation of mental disorder in Huntington's disease: a retrospective case record study of disease progression. *Acta Psychiatrica Scandinavica* 83, 53–60.

Pritchard, C., Zhu, N., Zuo, J., Bull, L., Pericak-Vance, M. A., Vance, J. M., Roses, A. D., Milatovich, A., Francke, U., Cox, D. R. & Myers, R. M. (1992). Recombination of 4p16 DNA markers in an unusual family with Huntington's disease. *American Journal of Human Genetics* 50, 1218–1230.

Propping, P. (1983). Genetic disorders presenting as schizophrenia: Karl Bonhoeffer's early review of the psychoses in the light of medical genetics. *Human Genetics* 65, 1–10.

Reed, T. E. & Chandler, J. H. (1958). Huntington's chorea in Michigan. 1. Demography and genetics. *American Journal of Human Genetics* 10, 201–225.

Robins, L. N., Helzer, J. E., Weissman, M. M., Overschel, H., Gruenberg, E., Burke, J. & Regier, A. D. (1984). Lifetime prevalence of specific psychiatric disorders in three sites. *Archives of General Psychiatry* 41, 949–958.

Rosenbaum, D. (1941). Psychosis with Huntington's chorea. *Psychiatric Quarterly* 15, 93–99.

Sambrook, J., Fritsch, E. & Maniatis, T. (1989). *Molecular Cloning: A Laboratory Manual*, 2nd edn. Cold Spring Harbor Laboratory Press: New York.

Saugstad, L. & Ødegård, O. (1986). Huntington's chorea in Norway. *Psychological Medicine* 16, 39–48.

Shepherd, M. & Sartorius, N. (1974). Personality disorder and the International Classification of Diseases. *Psychological Medicine* 4, 141–146.

Shields, J. (1978). The genetics of schizophrenia. In *Schizophrenia: Towards a New Synthesis* (ed. J. K. Wing), pp. 53–87. Academic Press: London.

Slater, E. & Cowie, V. (1971). *The Genetics of Mental Disorders*. Oxford University Press: London.

Snell, R. G., Lazarou, L., Youngman, S., Quarrell, O. W. J., Wasmuth, J. J., Shaw, D. J. & Harper, P. (1989). Linkage disequilibrium in Huntington's disease: an improved localisation for the gene. *Journal of Medical Genetics* 26, 673–675.

Stevens, D. L. (1976). Huntington's chorea: a demographic, genetic and clinical study. M.D. thesis, University of London.

Strachan, T. (1992). Analysing human DNA. In *The Human Genome*. (ed. A. P. Read and T. Brown), pp. 62–64. Bios Scientific Publishers: Oxford.

Streletzki, F. (1961). Psychosen in Verlauf der Huntingtonschen chorea unter besonderer Benachrichtigung der Wahnbildungen. *Archiv für Psychiatrie und Zeitschrift für der gesamte Neurologie* 202, 202–214.

Sydenham, T. (1848–1850). *The Entire Works of Thomas Sydenham*. Sydenham Society: London.

Tamir, A., Whittier, J. & Korenyi, C. (1969). Huntington's chorea: a sex difference in psychopathological symptoms. *Diseases of the Nervous System* 30, 103.

Thielmann, J., Kannini, S., Shiang, R., Robbins, C., Quarrell, O., Huggins, M., Hendrick, A., Weber, B., Collins, C., Wasmuth, J., Buetow, K., Murray, J. & Hayden, M. (1989). Non-random association between alleles detected at D4S95 and D4S98 and the Huntington's disease gene. *Journal of Medical Genetics*, 26, 676–681.

Walker, D. A., Harper, P. S., Wells, C. E. C., Tyler, A., Davies, K & Newcombe, R. G. (1981). Huntington's chorea in South Wales. *Clinical Genetics* 19, 213–221.

Wallace, D. C. (1972). Huntington's chorea in Queensland: a not uncommon disease. *Medical Journal of Australia* 1, 299–307.

Wallace, D. C. & Parker, N. (1973). Huntington's chorea in Queensland: the most recent story. In *Advances in Neurology* (ed. A. Barbeau, T. N. Chase and G. W. Poulson), vol. I. pp. 223–226. Raven Press: New York.

Wasmuth, J. J., Hewitt, J., Smith, B., Allard, D., Haines, J. L., Skarecky, D., Partlow, E. & Hayden, M. R. (1988). A highly polymorphic marker linked to the Huntington's disease gene. *Nature* 322, 734–736.

Wendt, G. G., Landzettel, H. J. & Unterreiner, I. (1959). Das Erkrankungsalter bei der Huntingtonschen Chorea. *Acta Genetica* 9, 18–32.

Wing, J. K., Cooper, J. & Sartorius, M. (1974). Measurement and Classification of Psychiatric Symptoms; *an Instruction Manual for the PSE and CATEGO Program*. Cambridge University Press: London.

World Health Organization (1978). *Mental Disorders: Glossary and Guide to Their Classification in Accordance with the Ninth Revision of the International Classification of Diseases*. WHO: Geneva.

Youngman, S., Sarfarazi, M., Bucan, M., MacDonald, M., Smith, B., Zimmerman, M., Gilliam, C., Frischauf, A., Wasmuth, J. J. & Gusella, J. (1989). A new marker D4S90 is located terminally on the short arm of chromosome 4, close to the Huntington's disease gene. *Genomics* 5, 802–809.